Skinny Bitch

Skinny Bitch

*A no-nonsense, tough-love guide for
savvy girls who want to stop eating crap
and start looking fabulous!*

by Rory Freedman and Kim Barnouin

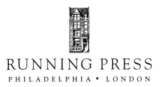

Running Press
PHILADELPHIA • LONDON

31 30 29 28 27 26 25 24 23 22 21
Library of Congress Control Number 2005901966

ISBN-13: 978-0-7624-2493-1
ISBN-10: 0-7624-2493-1

Cover and interior designed by Maria Taffera Lewis
Edited by Nancy Armstrong
Typography: Bauer Bodoni and Dutch 801

This book may be ordered by mail from the publisher.
Please include $2.50 for postage and handling.
But try your bookstore first!

Running Press Book Publishers
2300 Chestnut Street
Philadelphia, Pennsylvania 19103

Visit us on the web!
www.runningpress.com
www.skinnybitch.net

Contents

Acknowledgments 7

Introduction 10

Chapter 1: Give It Up 11

Chapter 2: Carbs: The Truth 22

Chapter 3: Sugar is the Devil 27

Chapter 4: The Dead, Rotting, Decomposing
    Flesh Diet 39

Chapter 5: The Dairy Disaster 55

Chapter 6: You Are What You Eat 65

Chapter 7: The Myths and Lies About Protein 84

Chapter 8: Pooping 89

Chapter 9: Have No Faith: Governmental Agencies
    Don't Give a Shit About Your Health 92

Chapter 10: Don't Be a Pussy 115

Chapter 11: Let's Eat 140

Chapter 12: FYI 177

Chapter 13: Use Your Head 184

Afterword 192

Recommended Reading 193

Sources Consulted 199

Endnotes 215

For Tony Robbins and Dr. Wayne Dyer,
with much love and appreciation.
It is because of your work that this book exists.

And for all the truth-speakers and seekers who have made
the world a better place while dramatically influencing our lives:
We thank you and honor all that you have done
and continue to do in the name of what is right.

Namastè.

Acknowledgments

It is with the utmost gratitude that we thank Lyssie Lakatos, Tammy Lakatos-Shames, Talia Cohen, Laura Dail, Jennifer Kasius, Maria Taffera Lewis, and Greg Jones for bringing this book to life. With awe, we acknowledge the editing brilliance of Nancy Armstrong, especially, but also the keen eyes of Meri Freedman and Dr. Amy Joy Lanou. A heartfelt thanks to our dream-team: Sam Caggiula, Seta Bedrossian, Allison Binder, and Scott Palmason for leading us above and beyond.

For your kind and patient help, we sincerely thank Matt Green, Bruce Friedrich, Holly Sternberg, Mark Gold, Kristina Johnson, Sara Chenoweth, Harold Brown, Ryan Zinn, Michele Simon, Talia Berman, Danielle Simon, Wayne Pacelle, Jay and Wendy Baxter, and Shaun Zaken. We are honored by the generous contributions of C. David Coates, Christine Hoza Farlow, D.C., and Tim VanOrden and cannot thank you enough.

Rory:

Kim, my partner in crime, I cannot imagine the existence I'd be leading if we never met. Thank you for changing the course of my life and enlightening me with your glow. You had me at hello.

It is with true adoration that I thank Tracy Silverman, who started me on this path, Lauren Silverman, who inspired me to commit to it more fully, Jesse Hildebrandt, for enabling me to do so, and my magical friends who made the journey by my side: Sue Foley, Todd and Lisa Adamek, Nora Ariffin, Emily Ashba, Dave Feeney, Fara Horowitz, Jill Iacuzzo, Jessica Jonas, Margaret Klinger, Denise Kunisch, Lisa Leder, Chris Lucia, Julie Lundberg, Kerri Meyers, Lori Morgen, Luke Orefice, Michelle Pappas, Andrea Pendas, Brian and MC Permenter, Jackie Poper, Randie Rolantz, Christine Santoro, Kim Snowden, Nora Stein, Louie and Christine Tibolla, Susan Weinberg, and all my PR pals who are too numerous to name.

To my grandmothers, Florence Freedman and Frances Levine, thank you for your inexhaustible supplies of love and faith. For your endless enthusiasm and loving encouragement, I thank my sister and brother-in-law, Lesley and Tim Bailey. Most of all, my parents, Rick and Meri Freedman— it is with an overflowing heart that I thank you for a lifetime of your unwavering support and love.

Kim:

My amazing friend and business partner, Rory,
without you none of this would be happening. I thank God every day
that we met and shared the same dream. We leapt
and the net appeared. Thank you for leaping with me.

Keesha Whitehurst Frederickson, I am so glad you are a part
of my life. Thank you for all the laughter and love,
and for being so special.

To all my other friends who honor me
with their day-to-day presence, I thank you.

A million thanks to my wonderful parents,
Richard and Linda Robinson, who believed in me and cheered me
on through the hard times and the good times.

To Jeri, Chrissy, Amanda, Melissa, Alex, and Elliot: I love you!

And last but not least, my love: my husband, Stephane.
There are not enough words in any language to express my love for
you. I am so grateful for your never-ending patience,
constant faith, pure love, and undying support.
I feel so blessed to be traveling through this life with you.
Je T'aime.

Introduction

A re you sick and tired of being fat? Good. If you can't take one more day of self-loathing, you're ready to get skinny. You don't need a degree in biology to get skinny. You don't need to starve yourself to get skinny. You don't need to spend all day at the gym to get skinny. You just need to smarten up and use your head. Really. It is that simple. We have been so brainwashed by fad diets, magazine articles, and advertising that we have forgotten how to think for ourselves.

Skinny Bitch delivers the truth about food, so that you can make intelligent and educated decisions for yourself. This knowledge will empower you to become a skinny bitch.

This is not a diet. This is a way of life. A way to enjoy food. A way to feel healthy, clean, energized and pure. It's time to reclaim your mind and body. It's time to strut your skinny ass down the street like you're in an episode of *Charlie's Angels* with some really cool song playing in the background. It's time to prance around in a thong like you rule the world. It's time to get skinny.

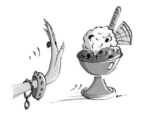

Chapter 1

Give It Up

O kay. Use your head. You need to get healthy if you want to get skinny. Healthy = skinny. Unhealthy = fat. The first thing you need to do is give up your gross vices. Don't act surprised! You cannot keep eating the same shit and expect to get skinny. Or smoke. So don't even try some pathetic excuse like, "But if I quit smoking, I'll gain weight." No one wants to hear it. Cigarettes are for losers. They are so 1989 and totally uncool. Not only do they screw up your whole body chemistry, but they also kill your taste buds. It's no wonder you eat shit and garbage. Smoking's out. Give it up.

Of course it's easier to socialize after you've had a few drinks. But being a fat pig will hinder you, sober or drunk. And habitual drinking equals fat-pig syndrome. Beer is for frat boys, not skinny bitches. It makes you fat, bloated, and farty. Why do you think when kids go away to college they gain the "freshman fifteen"? Beer, duh. Alcohol isn't any better. It raises the level of hydrochloric acid in your stomach, wreaking havoc on the digestive process. If you suffer from poor digestion, then your food will not pass through your body properly. Hence, bloated fat-pig syndrome. To make matters worse, some alcohol (and non-organic wines) still contains urethane, a cancer-causing chemical.[1] To boot, both beer and alcohol jack up your blood-sugar levels, which is bad for your bod. And don't kid yourself: When you have a hangover, you're bound to eat shit all day long. Trade your booze for organic red wine produced without sulfites. (Sulfites are additives—used in food and wine—to extend shelf life and fight bacteria growth. Asthma and allergic reactions can be triggered by sulfites. Even if wine is organic, that doesn't mean it is produced without sulfites. Read the label; it should say "No Sulfites Added" or "NSA." Frey Vineyards makes organic, sulfite-free wines.) This magical elixir— organic red wine with NSA—is rich in cancer-fighting antioxidants, can reduce risk of stroke, helps thin the blood, and has flavonoids, which lower cholesterol. Yes, organic red wine is good for you. No, you should not drink a bottle by yourself every day. Alcohol abuse can cause infertility, cancer, infectious diseases, cardiovascular disease, shrinking of the cerebral cortex, and alter brain-cell function. If you need help quitting drinking, call the Alcoholics Anonymous World Headquarters at (212) 870-3400 to find an AA meeting near you, or visit www.alcoholics-anonymous.org.

Brace yourselves, girls: Soda is liquid Satan. It is the devil. It is garbage. There is nothing in soda that should be put into your body. For starters, soda's high levels of phosphorous can increase calcium loss from the body, as can its sodium and caffeine. [Cousens, *Conscious Eating*, 475] You know what this means—bone loss, which may lead to osteoporosis. And the last time we checked, sugar, found in soda by the boatload, does not make you skinny! Now don't go patting yourself on the back if you drink diet soda. That stuff is even

Skinny Bitch

worse. Aspartame (an ingredient commonly found in diet sodas and other sugar-free foods) has been blamed for a slew of scary maladies, like arthritis, birth defects, fibromyalgia, Alzheimer's, lupus, multiple sclerosis, and diabetes.[2] When methyl alcohol, a component of aspartame, enters your body, it turns into formaldehyde. Formaldehyde is toxic and carcinogenic (cancer-causing).[3] Laboratory scientists use formaldehyde as a disinfectant or preservative. They don't fucking *drink* it. Perhaps you have a lumpy ass because you are preserving your fat cells with diet soda. The Food and Drug Administration (FDA) has received more complaints about aspartame than any other ingredient to date.[4] Want more bad news? When aspartame is paired with carbs, it causes your brain to slow down its production of serotonin.[5] A healthy level of serotonin is needed to be happy and well balanced. So drinking soda can make you fat, sick, and unhappy.

Unless you're from Mars, you've heard about the "eight glasses of water a day" thing. If you're filling up on 16 ounces of liquid Satan at a time, chances are you're not getting your 64 ounces of water a day. Water is vital for keeping your body clean and detoxified. It literally flushes out all the shit and toxins your body stores from your horrendous diet. You might be fat because you don't poop enough. Drinking lots of water can help with the elimination process. If the taste of water bores you, try jazzing up the flavor with a slice of lemon or lime, or, if you're feeling sassy, toss in a strawberry or raspberry. Say goodbye to soda and hello to a sweet ass.

"Don't talk to me until I've had my morning coffee." Uhm . . . *pathetic*! Coffee is for pussies. Think about how widely accepted it has become that people *need* coffee to wake up. You should not *need* anything to wake up. If you can't wake up without it, it's because you are either addicted to caffeine, sleep deprived, or a generally unhealthy slob. It may seem like the end of the world to give up your daily dose, especially if you rely on Starbucks as a good place to meet men. But it's not heroin, girls, and you'll learn to live without it. Caffeine can cause headaches, digestive problems, irritation of the stomach and bladder, peptic ulcers, diarrhea, constipation, fatigue, anxiety, and depression. It affects every organ system, from the nervous system to the skin. Caffeine raises stress hormone levels, inhibits important enzyme systems that are responsible for cleaning the body, and sensitizes nerve reception sites.[6] One study even links caffeine to an increased susceptibility to diabetes.[7] But don't go grabbing for the decaf. Coffee, whether regular or decaf, is highly acidic.[8] Acidic foods cause your body to produce fat cells, in order to keep the acid away from your organs.[9] (Please, do not link this acid issue to citrus and other fruits. We discuss this in depth later on page 38.) So coffee equals fat cells. P.S. It also makes your breath smell like ass. Furthermore, coffee beans, like other crops, are grown with chemical pesticides. One insecticide, D-D-7, has been banned in the United States, but is still used by other countries from which we import coffee beans.[10] So every single morning, you are starting your day with a dose of poison. Add sugar or other artificial sweeteners, top it off with milk or cream, and you'll be fat forever. If you enjoy an occasional cup of coffee, fine. But if you need it, give it up.

A much better way to start the day is with a cup of caffeine-free herbal tea—organic, of course. Decaffeinated green tea is like a wonder drug. Its anti-aging and antibacterial qualities are as renowned as its reputation for fighting cancer, combating allergies, and lowering blood pressure. Go to a coffeehouse, if you must. Just get a decaf organic herbal tea instead of coffee. Miss your caffeine jolt? Get a fresh-squeezed organic juice for an instant jumpstart. Once you are rid of your caffeine addiction, you will get totally high from fresh-squeezed juice.

Junk food will never go away. It becomes more alluring by the minute with laboratory-developed aromas, artificial flavors, chemical food colors, toxic preservatives, and heart-stopping hydrogenated oils. We know these are all impossible to resist, but no one ever got skinny on junk food. Use your head. Candy bars, potato chips, and ice cream taste like heaven, of course. But they will pitch a tent on your hips and camp out all year. Not only are they bogged down with saturated fats, sugars, hydrogenated oils, calories, and cholesterol, but they also contain enough chemical residues to put hair on your chest. Ever heard of butylated hydroxyamisole (BHA) or butylated hydroxytoluene (BHT)? Most people haven't, even though these chemical preservatives are either put in food or into the packaging.[11] The FDA doesn't require companies to divulge the presence of these beauties if they are used in packaging, though they can come into contact with the food you're eating. So your junk food has a shelf life of twenty-two years and will probably outlive your fat, sorry ass. Now before you decide you're so smart because you only buy fat-free snacks, get a hold of yourself. Whenever you see the words "fat-free" or "low-fat," think of the words "chemical shit storm." Read the ingredients. Do you really think sugar or hydrogenated oils or eggs or milk won't make you fat? Sober up, asshole. By the way, sugar, like coffee, creates an acidic environment in your body.[12] You just learned that acidic foods cause your body to produce fat cells. So you do the math: sugar = fat. If you'd drag your cankles to a health food store, you'd find aisle after aisle of "acceptable junk food." Guilt-free garbage that tastes so good, you'll do naked cartwheels around your living room. We are not saying you have to give up junk food to get skinny. You just have to trade your old junk food for new junk food. In Chapter 11, we provide an "acceptable junk food" list that'll make your nipples hard.

Are you a pill popper? Do you reach for over-the-counter medicine for every sniffle, sneeze, ache, and pain? Toughen up. Our bodies, when properly cared for, function as perfect machines. Our brains tell us when something is wrong by giving us pain or discomfort. When we pop pills to rid this "dis-ease," we are masking the symptoms without resolving the problem. Every time you take medicine, you interfere with your body's natural ability to heal itself. You are alleviating those intelligent responses that alert you to a problem, and sending false signals to your brain. If you have a headache, you might be tired, dehydrated, or suffering from a minor food allergy. Most likely, your body is having an adverse reaction to the unhealthy crap you're eating. Taking two aspirin is not the answer. If your nose is running, your body is trying to rid itself of something through your snot. But you, drama queen, take cold medicine to stop your booger flow. Now you've gone and fucked up everything. Medicine is made of chemicals. Never mind that the Food and Drug Administration gives meds their stamp of approval. They also allow the use of aspartame. Use your own damn brain. Do you think putting *chemicals* in your body is good for you? Every medicine comes complete with a list of side effects. That means that taking medicine will make you feel better for the moment, but will fuck up something else in your body. Yeah, getting cramps totally sucks. It's supposed to. Every month you endure cramps (without medication), you are preparing for the physical pain of childbirth. So suck it up. Stop interfering with Mother Nature.

(Obviously, if you are on prescribed medication, you need to consult a physician before discontinuing it.)

Give up the notion that you can be sedentary and still lose weight. You need to exercise, you lazy shit. Eating properly will dramatically improve your health, body, and all aspects of your life. But you've still gotta move your ass. Anyone with a brain can do the math: When done in conjunction with a good diet, exercise will make you lose weight faster than healthy eating alone. You don't need to spend seven days a week at the gym. In fact, you shouldn't, because too much exercise is bad for you. It can lead to dehydration, arthritis, osteoporosis, and injuries like strains, sprains, and fractures. Over-exercising can also cause low body-fat levels, which can disrupt the menstrual cycle and cause reproductive problems.[13] You want to be a Skinny Bitch, not a scrawny bitch. Twenty minutes of cardiovascular a day, five days a week, is a good starting point. Then, after a couple of weeks, kick it up a notch. Depending on your fitness goals, you can increase your cardiovascular workout or add strength training to your routine. Aim for working out in the morning, if you can. When we exercise, our elevated heart rates and deep breathing cause our "bodyminds" to enter a fat-burning mode that can last throughout the day.[14] Regardless of what time you work out, you'll soon become addicted to exercising. When we are active enough to break a sweat, our brains release endorphins and feel-good opiates. Exercise burns fat and calories, improves circulation, regulates crapping, defines muscles, builds strength, and detoxifies the body through sweating. Plus, working out tends to keep our junk food cravings and elephant appetites at bay. It's a win-win. Work out.

Chapter 2

Carbs: The Truth

N ever before has the United States seen such a ridiculous diet trend as the "low-carb" phenomenon. Every restaurant, grocery store, and fast-food chain caters to this utter nonsense. Even soda and beer companies have spent millions developing and marketing low-carb drinks. Everyone has jumped on the bandwagon, hoping to capitalize on the trend, whether it is healthy or not. Not.

Carbohydrates are compounds made up of carbon, hydrogen,

and oxygen, and they are *vital* for providing energy for our bodies and brains. Without them, we would be comatose zombies. When we eat food, our bodies turn the carbohydrates into glucose for immediate energy and the rest is stored as glycogen for reserves.

Yet all carbs are not created equal. There are two types: simple and complex. Simple carbohydrates suck and are as nutritionally beneficial as toilet paper. They are mostly made up of sugar, which releases too quickly, almost violently, into our bodies, causing "sugar highs" and then "crashes." This tends to leave us feeling hungry, so we eat more. On the other hand, complex carbohydrates are comprised of starch and fiber and release gradually, providing a steady source of energy. They make us feel full and satisfied and are easily broken down to release their energy. Shitty simple carbohydrates include white flour, white pasta (durum semolina), white rice, and white sugar. These are the bad boys that give all carbs a bad reputation. For some asinine reason, food manufacturers decided that we wouldn't buy their products unless they were white and soft. So they took natural grains, like brown rice and whole wheat, and stripped away all their nutrients, vitamins, and minerals to achieve the color and texture change. This refining process totally

compromises the nutritional integrity of the food—all for appearances. So companies then add these nutrients back into their
refined, milled foods and use terms like "enriched" or "fortified."
But there's no use trying to fool with Mother Nature. Our bodies
cannot absorb these added-in minerals with the same ease.[15]
Tragically, most cereals, pastas, rice, bagels, breads, cookies,
muffins, cakes, and pastries have been bastardized in this manner.
Pay attention to how your body feels when you eat these foods.
Chances are you'll notice moderate to severe mood swings and
energy surges and losses.

Fear not. There are so many complex carbohydrates (Mother
Nature is generous) that you'll never miss the simple shit. Bask in
the glory of potatoes, yams, sweet potatoes, barley, corn, brown
rice, beans, hummus, lentils, quinoa (a grain, pronounced KEEN-
wa), millet, and pasta made from brown rice, whole wheat, or
vegetables. Bionaturae, Ancient Harvest, Eddie's Spaghetti,
Lundberg Farms, Westbrae, Pastariso, and DeBoles Organic all
carry these "good carb" pastas. Relish the beauty of breads and
cookies and muffins made from whole wheat and other whole
grains. (Whole grains are any that haven't been bleached, stripped,

or refined and still possess all the nutrients from the original grain.)
Food For Life has an amazing line of whole and sprouted grain
breads, and Pacific Bakery and French Meadow Bakery carry
organic breads that aren't too shabby, either. Don't forget the
bounty of vegetables and fruits—complex carbs that supply the
body with vitamins, minerals, and fiber.

Yeah, you heard us—fruit. Eat it. The most irritating thing about
the low-carb craze is the resistance to eating fruit. Fruit is, quite pos-
sibly, the most perfect food in existence. It is unique in that it barely
requires any work to be digested. High in enzymes, it effortlessly
passes through the body, supplying carbohydrates, fiber, vitamins,
minerals, fatty acids, amino acids, and cancer-fighting tannins and
flavonoids. Because it is made up of mostly water, fruit hydrates the
body and aids in cleansing, detoxifying, and eliminating.

Best-selling *Fit for Life* authors Harvey and Marilyn Diamond
found that fruit best serves our bodies when eaten alone because it
is so easily and quickly digested. When we eat fruit with other
foods, it cannot pass through our bodies as quickly. So it rots and
ferments in our stomachs. This can cause burping, bloating, and
heartburn. To combat this, the Diamonds recommend eating fruit

on an empty stomach, first meal of the day, and waiting thirty minutes before eating anything else.[16] (We know this will be tough for some people, and it's okay if you aren't ready to tackle this challenge yet. It's just an ideal to aim for.)

So shout it from the rooftops until every one of your dumb-ass, misinformed friends hears: YOU CAN EAT BREAD AND FRUIT!

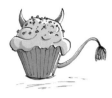

Chapter 3

Sugar is the Devil

W e all know how difficult it is to stay away from sugar. But if you don't exorcise this demon from your diet, you will never be a skinny bitch. Take a look around your kitchen and become aware of all the places the devil is lurking. Probably in places you wouldn't ever expect to find "him." Read the ingredients of your breakfast cereals, breads, crackers, junk foods, everything. Sugar is like crack, and food manufacturers know that if they add it to their products, you'll keep coming back for more.

What is this evil entity? In its simplest form, it is the juice from a sugar cane plant. A plant—that seems benign, right? And it is, in moderation, ingested in its raw, simplest form. But all the enzymes, fiber, vitamins, and minerals are destroyed during the refining process.[17] First, the cane is pressed to extract the juice. Then, the juice is boiled so that it will thicken and crystallize. Next, it is centrifuged, or spun, to remove the syrup. After that, the sugar is washed and filtered to remove any nonsugar materials and to decolorize it. (By the way, sugar filters are commonly made of charred animal bones. Nasty.) Finally, the sugar is dried and packaged. So you see, refined sugar has no nutritional value. And it's usually in foods that contain gobs of fat, lots of useless calories, and loads of cholesterol. So, you become addicted to foods (because they contain sugar) that have a large amount of fat, saturated fat, hydrogenated oils, and calories. Refined sugar, a simple carbohydrate, has been linked to hypoglycemia, yeast overgrowth (check your undies), a weakened immune system, hyperactivity, attention deficit disorder, enlargement of the liver and kidneys, increase of uric acid in the blood, mental and emotional disorders, dental cavi-

ties, and an imbalance of neurotransmitters in the brain.[18] In addition, refined sugars make you *fat*. Excess amounts are stored in the
liver as glycogen. But when the liver is too full, the excess amounts
are returned to the bloodstream as fatty acids.[19] Guess where those
end up? Hips, stomach, thighs, and ass.

The sugar industry is big business in America. The United States
is the largest supplier of sugar-laden foods in the world. It's not
enough to poison our own citizens. We have to fuck up the rest of
the world, too, for a dime.

High fructose corn syrup is another badass that finds its way into
tons of foods. Manufacturers love its versatility and put it in nearly
everything: juice, soda, beer, yogurt, energy bars, cookies, candies,
breads, even frozen goods. High fructose corn syrup is processed
more than sugar and is even sweeter. But it's a friend of the farmer
because it's so cheap to produce. Like refined sugar, it has a negative, dramatic effect on our blood-sugar levels. According to studies
conducted by the *American Journal of Clinical Nutrition,* diabetes
and obesity are directly linked to eating refined sugar and high
fructose corn syrup.[20]

We aren't telling you to give up cookies for the rest of your lives;

we certainly don't want to start a riot. We're simply suggesting that you substitute natural, healthier alternatives for refined sugar. At the top of the list is agave nectar or syrup. This high-nutrient sweetener can actually be beneficial to your health. It doesn't contain any processing chemicals, and the raw version (completely unprocessed) contains vitamins and minerals. Because it absorbs slowly into the bloodstream, agave nectar doesn't have a significant impact on blood-sugar levels. It can be used in place of sugar in any product or recipe.

Stevia, another winner, is derived from a plant found in Paraguay. The Japanese have been using this wonder sweetener for decades, South Americans for centuries. In fact, it is used by hundreds of millions of people around the world to balance blood-sugar levels, reduce cravings for sweets, and aid in digestion. Additionally, it is known for its antimicrobial properties (it inhibits the growth of bacteria). Unfortunately, however, it is the most unrecognized sweetener in the United States. This natural, herbal sweetener contains no calories, has no glycemic index (meaning it won't alter blood sugar), and is even safe for diabetics. But for reasons unknown to intelligent species everywhere, the Food and Drug

Administration won't approve Stevia for use in food products.[21] Maybe they are sleeping with the sugar industry.

Other good substitutes for refined sugar include evaporated cane juice, Sucanat, brown rice syrup, barley malt syrup, Rapadura sugar, Turbinado sugar, raw sugar, beet sugar, date sugar, maple syrup, molasses, and blackstrap molasses. (Some companies add lard to maple syrup or molasses to reduce foaming, so be sure you are buying 100 percent pure, organic products.) Don't shit and piss yourselves, but all of these natural sweeteners possess one or more of the following health benefits: enzymes, calcium, iron, potassium, protein, the B vitamins, magnesium, chromium, fiber, and folic acid. Some even contain complex carbohydrates.[22] We're not saying you should eat naturally sweetened cupcakes three meals a day. We're just saying that you *can* have your cake and eat it. Just use your head regarding the amount of sweets you consume.

A drum roll, please, for a few of our favorite sweets: Uncle Eddie's vegan cookies, Tropical Source or Terra Nostra chocolate bars, Oreo knock-offs by Back to Nature or Country Choice, organic Fig Newmans, and all the cookies by the Sun Flour Baking Co. and the Alternative Baking Co.

Now that you've heard the good news about natural sweeteners, it's time to give up the all the bad ones. Obviously, refined sugar is bad for you, as is high fructose corn syrup. And in case you had your head up your ass during Chapter 1, STOP EATING AND DRINKING PRODUCTS THAT CONTAIN ASPARTAME! This includes diet sodas and sugar-free foods that have NutraSweet or Equal.

When aspartame was put before the FDA for approval, it was denied *eight* times. G.D. Searle, founder of aspartame, tried to get FDA approval in 1973. Clearly, he wasn't bothered by reports from neuroscientist Dr. John Olney and researcher Ann Reynolds (hired by Searle himself) that aspartame was dangerous. Dr. Martha Freeman, a scientist from the FDA Division of Metabolic and Endocrine Drug Products, declared, "The information submitted for review is inadequate to permit a scientific evaluation of clinical safety." Freeman recommended that until the safety of aspartame was proven, marketing the product should not be permitted. Alas, her recommendations were ignored. Somehow, in 1974, Searle got approval to use aspartame in dry foods. However, it wasn't smooth sailing from there. In 1975, the FDA put together a task force to review Searle's testing methods. Task force team leader Phillip

Brodsky said he "had never seen anything as bad as Searle's testing" and called test results "manipulated." Before aspartame
actually made it into dry foods, Olney and attorney and consumer
advocate Jim Turner filed objections against the approval.[23]

In 1977, the FDA asked the U.S. attorney's office to start grand
jury proceedings against Searle for "knowingly misrepresenting
findings and concealing material facts and making false statements
in aspartame safety tests." Shortly after, the U.S. attorney leading
the investigation against Searle was offered a job by the law firm
that was representing Searle. Later that same year, he resigned as
U.S. attorney and withdrew from the case, delaying the grand jury's
investigation. This caused the statute of limitations on the charges
to run out, and the investigation was dropped. *And* he accepted the
job with Searle's law firm.[24] Stunning.

In 1980, a review by the Public Board of Inquiry set up by the
FDA determined that aspartame should not be approved. The
board said it had "not been presented with proof of reasonable cer-
tainty that aspartame is safe for use as a food additive." In 1981, new
FDA Commissioner Arthur Hull Hayes was appointed. Despite the
fact that three out of six scientists advised against approval, Hayes

decided to overrule the scientific review panel and allow aspartame into limited dry goods. In 1983, he got it approved for beverages, even though the National Soft Drink Association urged the FDA to delay approval until further testing could be done. That same year, Hayes left the FDA amid charges of impropriety. The Internal Department of Health and Human Services was investigating Hayes for accepting gratuities from FDA-regulated companies. He went to work as a consultant for Searle's public relations firm. Interesting. The FDA finally urged Congress to prosecute Searle for giving the government false or incomplete test results on aspartame.[25] However, the two government attorneys assigned to the case decided not to prosecute. Later, they went to work for the law firm that represented Searle. Fascinating. Despite recognizing ninety-two different symptoms that result from ingesting aspartame, the FDA approved it for use, without restriction, in 1996.[26] Brilliant.

So many people have been sickened from this shit that there are aspartame victim support groups. Some of the ninety-two aspartame side effects listed by the FDA include memory loss, nerve cell damage, migraines, reproductive disorders, mental confusion, brain lesions, blindness, joint pain, Alzheimer's, bloating, nervous system disorders, hair loss, food cravings, and weight gain.[27]

Aspartame is a $1 billion industry.[28] The National Justice League has filed a series of lawsuits against food companies using aspartame, claiming they are poisoning the public. In September 2004, a class action lawsuit was filed for $350 million against NutraSweet and the American Diabetics Association. Secretary of Defense Donald Rumsfeld is named in the suit for using political muscle to get aspartame approved by the FDA.[29]

NutraSweet and Equal contain aspartame. When ingested, one of aspartame's ingredients, methyl alcohol, converts into formaldehyde, a deadly neurotoxin.[30] In addition to aspartame, Equal contains the amino acid phenylalanine. Phenylalanine occurs naturally in the brain. But high levels can increase the chance of seizures and lead to depression and schizophrenia.[31] There is no lesser of the two evils. NutraSweet and Equal are both evil. Sweet & Low is no saint, either. It is an artificial sweetener that contains saccharin, a coal-tar compound.[32] Stay away.

Because we're having so much fun, let's bash the shit out of Splenda, one of the newer sweeteners. Splenda is made by chlorinating sugar, changing its molecular structure. The finished product is called sucralose. The makers of this poison tout its lack of calories and claim it's safe for diabetics. The FDA calls sucralose 98 percent pure. The other 2 percent contains small amounts of heavy metals, methanol, and arsenic.[33] Well, gee, at least it doesn't have calories. So what if it has a little arsenic? Sucralose has been found to cause diarrhea; organ, genetic, immune system, and reproductive damage; swelling of the liver and kidneys; and a decrease in fetal body weight.[34] What a splendid product! According to Dr. Joseph Mercola in Consumer Research magazine's article "The Potential Dangers of Sucralose," "There is no clear-cut evidence that sugar substitutes are useful in weight reduction. On the contrary, there is some evidence that these substances may stimulate appetite."[35]

Not only have multiple class action lawsuits been filed, but even the president of the National Sugar Association and the manufacturer of Equal are up in arms about Splenda. They each filed suit, claiming that Splenda manufacturers are misleading consumers into thinking the product is natural when it is "a highly processed chemical compound." Don't think that the giants behind artificial sweeteners and the sugar industry suddenly started caring about public health. Splenda's clever marketing is just totally screwing up their sales. But even executive director for the Center for Science in the Public Interest, Dr. Michael F. Jacobson, who normally criticizes The National Sugar Association, had to agree: "Advertising and labeling, whether for products that are healthful or unhealthful, should be truthful and not misleading." [36]

Clearly, artificial sweeteners and refined sugars are bad for many reasons. Here's one more. We have a delicate balancing act occurring in our bodies at all times—pH balance. Basically, everything we eat has its own pH balance. When food is digested, it leaves an acid or alkaline "ash" in the body, depending on the food's mineral content. Surprise, surprise: Artificial sweeteners are highly acid forming. (Coffee, excessive protein, meat, pasteurized dairy, refined sugars, and fatty foods are, too.)[37]

When our bodies get too acidic, we are much more prone to illness. Sometimes, we don't even know we're sick until it's too late. But we can notice mild maladies, like skin problems, allergies, headaches, colds, or yeast infections. Or, we can experience major trauma—severe damage to our thyroid gland, liver, and adrenal glands. If our pH balance becomes too acidic, our bodies will react to protect themselves. To neutralize the acid, they will take alkalizing minerals from our reserves. If our reserves are low, the body will withdraw minerals from our bones and muscles.[38] If that doesn't scare you, consider this: It is commonly believed that cancer cells thrive in acid environments.[39]

Now, logically, you would think that citrus fruits are acidic, but actually, when they enter the body, they are alkalizing. We know this goes against the "use your own head" idea because they seem like they'd be acidic. But they contain potassium and calcium, which are alkalizing minerals. They also have a high percentage of alkaline salts. Nearly all fruits, vegetables, and legumes are alkaline when they enter the body.[40] Other alkalizing foods are sea vegetables, miso, soybeans, and tofu.

Fruit, good. Natural sweeteners, good. Refined sugars, bad. Artificial sweeteners, bad. Any questions?

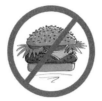

Chapter 4

The Dead, Rotting, Decomposing Flesh Diet

The Atkins diet. Hmm. Eat the flesh of dead cows, dead pigs, and dead chickens. Avoid fresh fruit. You are a total moron if you think the Atkins diet will make you thin. Or, you are a gluttonous pig who wants to believe you can eat cheeseburgers all day long and lose weight. Perhaps you weren't listening the first time: You need to get healthy if you want to be skinny! Eating carcasses all day while avoiding fruit is a recipe for disaster. Of course, if you stop eating refined carbohydrates, you will lose weight. That's the part of the Atkins Diet that actually works. However, most of the weight you lose is water weight. You see, when our bodies metabolize protein (found in high amounts in meat and dairy), nitrogen waste is released in the form of urea. Urea is toxic and must be passed out of the body through urine. So the high-protein diet isn't ridding your body of fat. It's just serving as a diuretic—making you pee more to flush out the toxic urea.[41] But whether you lose this piss weight initially is inconsequential. You will be a fat, unhealthy, bloated pig if you live this way.

Trendy diets like Atkins become popular for one reason: They hide behind scientific jargon that *seems* to make sense and allow you to eat unhealthy, fattening foods as long as you avoid carbs. You believe in these diets because you want to. Most Americans eat twice as much protein as necessary, which has sent obesity, heart disease, and cancer rates soaring over the past fifty years. When you eat large amounts of animal protein and saturated fats and do not eat whole grains, vegetables, and fresh fruits, there is no fiber to bind all of the toxins and fat together to be eliminated from your body. You will eventually do an incredible amount of harm to yourself. Your poor kidneys are in serious jeopardy of developing stones, aging prematurely, and failing altogether. They must work twice as hard to break down protein and remove waste. By the time your blood shows the effects, it will be too late to reverse the damage. Diabetics are in even worse trouble with a high-protein diet because they are already at a higher risk of kidney disease to begin with. In a study involving 1,500 patients with diabetes, most had lost more than half of their kidney function because of a high intake of animal protein.[42] Don't care about your kidneys and just want to lose weight? The American Cancer Society conducted a study over a ten-year period with nearly 80,000 people trying to lose weight. Participants who ate meat three times a week or more gained substantially more weight than participants who avoided meat and consumed more vegetables.[43] Studies published in *The Journal of Clinical Nutrition and The New England Journal of Medicine* stated that meat eaters are much more likely to be overweight than vegetarians.[44]

Before you start spouting off information you've been brainwashed with about evolution and the food chain, read on. Yes, humans have a high level of intelligence. Yes, we created weapons for hunting and fire for cooking. Yes, we found a way to mass-produce animals for consumption. However, if you study animals in the wild, you will note that they do not rely on anything other than their natural hunting ability, speed, strength, claws, teeth, and jaws. They have no tools or weapons. Now look at yourself. Look at your flimsy fingernails in comparison to an eagle's talons. Look at your flat, blunt teeth compared to a lion's fangs. Compare your speed and agility to that of a tiger. Compare the strength of your jaw to a wolf's. Imagine yourself trying to run after an animal, catch it, and kill it using your bare hands, fingernails, teeth, and jaws. Not only would you look ridiculous, but you'd probably get your ass kicked, too. And even if you were successful, envision yourself eating the kill without the aid of an oven and silverware.[45] Yes, the human brain allows us to stay removed from the process of hunting. But does this mean we are "evolved" and "intelligent" and should be eating animal flesh just because we can? Man's "intelligence" also created alcohol, cigarettes, and drugs. Should we drink, smoke, and use just because we can?

Many meat eaters credit eating meat for our evolution from

cavemen into what we are now. Even if this were the case and eating meat did help us to evolve, look at what we evolved *from*. We looked liked friggin' apes and had massive heads, strong jaws, and brute strength. Maybe back then we were supposed to eat meat. But the last time we checked, we aren't cavemen anymore.

The second we put food in our mouths, the digestion process begins, thanks to our saliva. Guess what? Our alkaline saliva is not meant to break down animal flesh; carnivores have acid saliva, perfectly designed for the task. And hydrochloric acid, essential for digesting carcass, is secreted in very small amounts in our stomachs. However, the stomachs of carnivores have ten times more hydrochloric acid than ours. Our enzymes, digestive tracts, and organs are all different from those found in carnivores. Like it or not, our kidneys, colon, and liver are ill-equipped to process animal flesh. Compared to carnivores, our intestines are very long, so food that doesn't get adequately processed becomes clogged in our intestines. Animals quickly pass food through their digestive systems, but we have food rotting, decomposing, and fermenting in our intestinal tracts and colons, hence the need for colonics (aka: enemas). You don't see many tigers getting colonics, do you? You do see them napping, though. Even though their bodies are designed to digest meat, animals generally sleep all day while doing so because it is such a taxing process. Genetically and structurally, we are designed to thrive on plant foods.[46] Whether it is "lean meat" or a "skinless chicken breast," animal fat is still animal fat. Don't be fooled by terms coined by the meat industry. Your body can't handle animal fat, so it settles like lumpy shit all over your ass, thighs, sides, arms, and stomach.

And then there are the gross, stomach-turning realities of the meat-production industry.

Of the ten billion animals slaughtered each year in America for human consumption, the vast majority of them come from factory farms. Factory farms that raise cattle, pigs, chickens, egg-laying hens, veal calves, or dairy cows have an enormous amount of animals in a very small space. There are no vast meadows or lush, green pastures. The animals are confined inside buildings, where they are literally packed in on top of each other. Egg-laying hens are crammed into cages so small, they are unable to open their wings, and their mangled feet actually grow around the wire mesh floors. This overcrowded, stressful environment causes chickens to peck at each other and factory farm workers, so the ends of their beaks are seared off their faces using a hot knife. Pigs and cows are imprisoned in stalls so small, they are unable to turn around or lie down comfortably. Cattle are subject to third-degree branding burns and having their testicles and horns ripped out. Pigs also suffer from branding and castration, in addition to the mutilation of their ears, tails, and teeth. They all live in the filth of their own urine, feces, and vomit with infected, festering sores and wounds. To keep animals alive in these unsanitary conditions, farmers must give them regular doses of antibiotics.

Half of all the antibiotics made in the United States each year are administered to farm animals, causing antibiotic resistance in the humans who eat them.[47] A study at the University of California-Berkeley linked eating beef to urinary tract infections (UTIs) in women. It just so happens that the most common infectious disease in women is UTIs.[48] You do the math.

For shits and giggles, we've compiled a partial list of what's in meat, poultry, seafood, and dairy: benzene hexachloride (BHC), chlordane, dichlorodiphenyltrichloroethane (DDT), dieldrin, dioxin, heptachlor, hexachlorobenzene (HCB), and lindane.[49] Perhaps that's why eating "meat" has been linked to obesity; cancer; liver, kidney, lung, and reproductive disorders; birth defects; miscarriages; and nervous system disorders.[50] American farmers started using chemical pesticides in the late 1800s and were initially thrilled with the results. However, it was eventually noticed that pesticides were killing those who were most exposed to them: farmers, field workers, and animals. In 1972, the Environmental Protection Agency banned DDT.[51] But the pesticides that followed were even worse. BHC is 19 times more carcinogenic than DDT, chlordane 4 times more, dieldrin 47 to 85 times more, HCB 23 times more, and heptachlor 15 to 30 times more. By the late 1980s, of the 450 endangered animal species, more than half were threatened with extinction. The government finally called for a ban on the production and use of other pesticides. But this didn't stop these pesticides from reaching our food supply. Companies were allowed to use up their enormous stockpiles of these pesticides by selling them to countries outside of America. (Apparently, it was acceptable to poison people and animals as long as they weren't American.) These countries used the pesticides on their crops, which were then imported into the United States.[52] Brilliant, huh? And, banned or not, once they have entered the soil or water, pesticides can still poison for decades.[53]

One widely used herbicide, glufosinate, whose residues have been found in U.S. waters and food supplies, causes hormonal and brain damage.[54] In his book, *Diet for a Poisoned Planet,* David Steinman reports that of all the toxic chemicals found in food, 95 to 99 percent come from meat, fish, dairy, and eggs.[55] He also reveals that many of the tests performed don't even detect many chemicals and pesticides. The Food and Drug Administration's own Total Diet Study found that bacon had 48 different pesticide residues, bologna and other luncheon meats had 102 different industrial pollutants and pesticides, fast food hamburgers had 113 residues, hot dogs had 123, and ground beef had 82 industrial chemical and pesticide residues, just to name a few.[56] In comparison, meat contains 14 times more pesticides than plant foods, and dairy has 5 times more pesticides than plant foods. The United States alone uses *one billion pounds* of pesticides every year on our food. That, our pathetic contamination sampling process, and our use of growth hormones has caused the European Economic Community to reject our meat exportations on numerous occasions.[57]

Many animals are even given arsenic-laced drugs.[58] Arsenic!

Chemical pesticides are often sprayed directly onto the skin of animals to ward off parasites, insects, rodents, and fungi. In addition, these animals are given food treated with pesticides. On factory farms, bigger is better. More meat, milk, and eggs mean more money for the farmers. So to grow them larger or have them produce more, animals are given steroids and growth hormones. But what is happening to the people who eat these fattened animals? Young girls are experiencing an early onset of puberty at epidemic proportions. Many scientists attribute this to all of the hormones in chicken, meat, and milk that are forced upon children. Basically, every time you consume factory-farmed chicken, beef, veal, pork, eggs, or dairy, you are eating antibiotics, pesticides, steroids, and hormones. This is worth repeating: *Every time you consume factory-farmed chicken, beef, veal, pork, eggs, or dairy, you are eating antibiotics, pesticides, steroids, and hormones.*

Now you might be thinking, "Who cares about all this pesticide-cancer shit? I just want to get skinny!" Ever been on The Pill and gained weight? Ever gained weight from having fertility treatments? Well, eating animals that are given hormones has the same effect as if you were taking these directly. According to Dr. Paula

Baillie-Hamilton, author of *The Body Restoration Plan,* antibiotics alone can account for weight gain in animals.[59] She also states that the toxic chemicals used in food production are fattening. Whether it's the pesticides used for growing crops or the chemicals given to animals to fatten them up, they alter the body's metabolism in a way that causes weight gain. Having studied animals and humans, she discovered that low doses of toxic chemicals increased appetite, slowed metabolism, decreased ability to burn stored fat, and reduced ability to exercise.[60] The FDA lists approximately 1,700 drugs approved for use in animal feed. Of these approved drugs, approximately 300 include "weight gain" in their description.[61] However, in their book *Animal Factories,* Jim Mason and Peter Singer disclose an estimate of 20,000 to 30,000 different drugs actually being used.[62]

We constantly hear the snobby declaration, "I don't eat any red meat. I just eat chicken." Well now you know: Chicken is just as bad for you as cow or pig. In fact, it might even be worse. According to the American *Journal of Epidemiology,* eating chicken (and fish) is linked to colon cancer. Researchers examined the eating habits of 32,000 men and women over a six-year period and then monitored emerging cancer cases for the next six years. "Among participants who generally avoided red meat but who ate white meat less than once per week, colon cancer risk was 55 percent higher than for those who avoided both kinds of meat. Those who had white meat at least once per week had more than three-fold higher colon cancer risk." [63] Researchers at the National Cancer Institute found grilled chicken to have high levels of heterocyclic amines, carcinogens that are formed when animal proteins are heated. With 480 nanograms of heterocyclic amines per gram, grilled chicken registered 15 times higher than beef.[64]

Do not be lulled into a false sense of security that our government keeps food safe. News of the avian influenza epidemic came and went, but this disease is very real and can run rampant in poultry flocks. And according to a survey by the National Research Council, one chicken processing plant had 90 percent of its poultry contaminated with salmonellosis.[65] Ninety fucking percent! Nasty.

Unfortunately, our waters aren't any better than our land. Yes, some fish contain essential fatty acids and vitamins, minerals, and protein. But you can easily get all these nutrients from flaxseeds; pumpkin, sesame, and sunflower seeds; nuts; soybeans; fruits; vegetables; leafy greens; soy products; and whole grains. Fish and other seafood contain high levels of contaminants from industrial and environmental pollutants, waste products, and pesticide residues from farms. Also present in fish and seafood are high levels of mercury and PCBs, which are well absorbed by the body. Other notables are BHC, chlordane, DDT, dieldrin, heptachlor, and dioxin.[66] These chemicals can cause neurotoxicity, which impairs a person's mental state and ability. The human body contains acetylcholine, a naturally occurring chemical that helps impulses pass from nerve to nerve. Once the impulse is passed, the chemical is no longer needed and is actually harmful if it remains. So our bodies produce an enzyme, cholinesterase, which rids us of the unwanted acetylcholine. Pesticides inhibit our ability to produce cholinesterase, which causes a buildup of the now-dangerous acetycholine.[67] Mercury, a suspected carcinogen, can alter immune function, raise blood pressure, cause blindness or paralysis, increase the chance of cardiac mortality, and is known to reduce fertility and virility.[68] It can also inflict permanent brain damage on fetuses, infants, and children.

Appetizing, huh? Have some mercury poisoning with your ahi tuna. How about some trichinosis with your pork? Don't forget a side of salmonella with your eggs or chicken. We certainly don't want to leave out an order of mad cow disease. Think about what you've been eating. What we call salmon, hamburger, steak, chicken, bacon, sausage, ham, roast beef, salami, bologna, turkey, hot dog, and duck are actually decomposing, rotting animal carcasses. *Bon appétit!*

Closing your eyes to the problem will not make it go away. You don't want to see it, but you'll *eat* it? So, yeah, if you want to get skinny, you've got to be a vegetarian—someone who doesn't eat dead animals or seafood. Quit whining. We weren't raised by hippie-crunchy-granola parents on vegetarian communes. Growing up, we both ate meat all day, every day. We scoffed at tofu and spit on vegetables. Really. Kim's addictions included such delicacies as corned beef hash, canned Vienna sausages, and daily Big Macs. Every single day in 1992, Rory ate a ham, egg, and cheese sandwich for breakfast, followed by a bacon double cheeseburger, fries, and a soda for lunch. Dinner was always a dead chicken, fish, cow, or pig. Now granted, we didn't give up meat just to get skinny. We both became vegetarians after learning about the treatment of farm animals. But we each noticed big changes in our minds, attitudes, health, moods, and asses when we gave up carcass. So before you say, "I could never give up meat," realize that nearly every single vegetarian on the planet said those same words. Then shut the fuck up, look at an inspirational picture of a skinny bitch, and clean out your freezer.

There are a ton of awesome, soy-based fake meat products on the market. Not only do they taste great, but soy has been lauded for lowering cholesterol, protecting against cancer, reducing the risk of heart attacks,[69] and helping the body to better utilize calcium. Phytoestrogens, found in soy, help protect women from breast cancer and can alleviate menopausal symptoms.[70] However, there are opponents to soy, who claim that it can negatively impact the thyroid, cause mineral deficiencies, and raise the risk of breast cancer. But according to health expert Dr. Andrew Weil, "There is still much to be learned about soy, but the majority of research so far has shown that it's a safe and nutritious food when eaten in reasonable amounts—about one or two daily servings."[71] We encourage you to think for yourself and make your own decision.

If you decide to eat soy products that imitate meat products, know that these foods may not taste exactly like the real thing. But once you get rid of your meat addiction, you'll be satisfied with the substitutes. You just need to spend a few weeks (and dollars) experimenting until you find the ones you like. Veggie burgers exist by the dozen. Health Is Wealth makes fake buffalo wings that taste so good, your pubes will fall out. Gardenburger's Flame-Grilled Chik'n is so amazing, you might have to kill yourself. Lightlife has a kick-ass line of "cold cuts" and fabulous "bacon." One amazing website is *www.vegieworld.com*. It is an Asian mail order company that not only sells fake chicken and meat, but has fake seafood, too. But you don't have to look far: Seek and ye shall find. We list lots of meatless wonders in Chapter 11. But remember, getting skinny means using your head. You must read all the ingredients and make sure there are *no* animal products in anything you buy. For the rest of your skinny life, every time you buy something that you will be swallowing, you must read the ingredients.

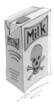

Chapter 5

The Dairy Disaster

G o suck your mother's tits. Go on. Suck your mother's tits. You think this is ridiculous? It is. Get ready to use your head.

When a woman gives birth, her body produces milk and she nurses her child.

Breast milk can grow an 8-pound newborn into a 24-pound toddler. Sounds pretty fattening, huh? It is. By design, it is intended to allow for the biggest growth spurt of a person's entire life. Breast milk alone can accommodate for a 300 percent weight gain in a twelve-month period. When her child is anywhere from 12 to 24 months old, a mother stops breast feeding. Her milk dries up. The child will never drink breast milk ever again.

Cows, like all mammals, are much the same. Their bodies produce milk only when they give birth. Contrary to popular belief, they do not need to be milked—ever. Their udders, like women's breasts, exist even when there is no milk in them. There is one major difference, however. Cows' milk, by design, grows a 90-pound calf into a 2,000-pound cow over the course of two years.[72] It allows calves to double their birth weight in forty-seven days and leaves their four stomachs feeling full. Sounds even more fattening than human milk, right? It is. It should be. Cows are bigger than humans. And the inner workings of their bodies are completely different than ours, which they should be. They are cows. We are humans. Duh.

Mammals need the enzyme lactase to digest lactose (the sugar found in dairy). However, between the ages of 18 months and 4 years, we lose 90 to 95 percent of this enzyme. The undigested lactose and the acidic nature of pasteurized milk encourage the growth of bacteria in our intestines.[73] All this contributes to a greater risk of cancer because cancer cells thrive in acidic conditions.[74]

Got mucus? Dairy products produce mucus, and often, the body will develop a cold or "allergies" to fight the dairy invasion.[75] Mother Nature is no fool. All species, including ours, have just what we need to get by. She did not intend for grownups to suck their mothers' tits. We don't need our mothers' milk as adults, just like grown cows don't need their mothers' milk anymore. We are the only species on the planet that drinks milk as adults. We are also the only species on the planet that drinks the milk of another species. We could be putting gorilla milk on our cereal or having zebra milk and cookies. Why cows' milk? Using the animal that produces the largest quantity of milk but is more easily housed than an elephant means more money for farmers. It has nothing to do with health or nutrition. Again, it all comes back to money. The dairy industry is a multibillion-dollar industry based on brilliant marketing and the addictive taste of milk, butter, and cheese. It has convinced most doctors, consumers, and government agencies that we *need* cows' milk. We have been told our whole lives, "You need milk to grow. Without milk, your bones will break. If you don't drink milk, you'll get osteoporosis. You need the calcium." *Bullshit*.

Researchers at Harvard, Yale, Penn State, and the National Insti-
tutes of Health have studied the effects of dairy intake on bones.
Not one of these studies found dairy to be a deterrent to osteoporosis.[76] On the contrary, a study funded by the National Dairy Council
itself revealed that the high protein content of dairy actually leaches
calcium from the body.[77] After looking at thirty-four published studies in sixteen countries, researchers at Yale University found that
the countries with the highest rates of osteoporosis—including the
United States, Sweden, and Finland—were those in which people
consumed the most meat, milk, and other animal foods.[78] Another
study showed that though 40 million American women have osteoporosis, only 250,000 African women have bone disease. In fact, of
the forty tribes in Kenya and Tanzania, only one—the Maasai—has
members suffering from osteoporosis. The Maasai, as it happens,
are a cattle-owning, milk-drinking tribe.[79]

Dairy products have been linked to a host of other problems,
too, including acne, anemia, anxiety, arthritis, attention deficit disorder, attention deficit hyperactivity disorder, fibromyalgia,
headaches, heartburn, indigestion, irritable bowel syndrome, joint
pain, osteoporosis, poor immune function,[80] allergies, ear infec-

tions, colic, obesity, heart disease, diabetes, autism, Crohn's disease, breast and prostate cancers,[81] and ovarian cancer.[82]

Harvey and Marilyn Diamond, authors of best-selling follow-up *Fit For Life II,* clearly state, "DAIRY PRODUCTS ARE DISEASE-PRODUCING. They're harmful. They *cause* suffering. They're the perfect thing to eat if you want to be sick and have a diseased body. The dietitians and nutritionists who are mouthpieces and cheerleaders for the dairy industry, telling you that dairy products are a good food, should hide their heads in shame—not only for leading the innocent to believe that dairy products are actually valuable, but also for failing to keep abreast of the field about which they are *supposed* to know something."

Yes, we are saying it is common knowledge in the medical research field that dairy is bad for you. Yes, we are saying that executives in the dairy industry are well aware of this fact but make claims that milk "does a body good." How do they get away with this? Easily. They spend hundreds of millions of dollars every year to market their products. And average consumers don't spend their time perusing medical journals, but they do read magazines and watch television.

What about medical doctors? Why do they believe that milk is beneficial? It is a sad fact that in this country, most doctors know almost nothing about nutrition. According to a Senate investigation, doctors receive *less than three hours* of nutritional training in medical school.[83] They have been duped like the rest of us.

Let's pretend for a moment that cows' milk is healthy for humans. Even if it were, by the time factory farms were done with it, it wouldn't be. Dioxin, one of the most toxic substances in the world, is often found in dairy products.[84] And remember, for factory farms, higher production means bigger profits. When you consume dairy products, you are ingesting the same antibiotics, pesticides, steroids, and hormones you would if you ate meat directly. Cows are injected with bovine growth hormone. Their udders, under normal conditions, would supply about ten pounds of milk a day. Greedy farmers have their cows producing up to a hundred pounds of milk a day! There is no gentle farmer milking the cow with a bucket between his feet. Cows are milked by machine; metal clamps are attached to the cows' sensitive udders. The udders become sore and infected. Pus forms. But the machines keep on milking, sucking the dead white blood cells into the milk.[85] How freaking gross is that? To get rid of all the bacteria and other shit, milk must be pasteurized. But pasteurization destroys beneficial enzymes and makes calcium less available without even killing all the viruses or bacteria. Hell, even radioactive particles are found in milk![86]

But don't the government and U.S. Department of Agriculture protect us from all this? Hell no. Sickeningly high levels of pesticides found in dairy meet government standards. Records from the Food and Drug Administration show that "virtually 100% of the cheese products produced and sold in the U.S. has detectable pesticide residues." [87]

Milk is not a reliable source of minerals. You get much higher levels of manganese, chromium, selenium, and magnesium from fruits and vegetables. Fruits and veggies are also high in boron, which helps lessen the loss of calcium through urine.[88] Consuming high amounts of dairy blocks iron absorption, contributing to iron deficiency.[89]

So do you need calcium by the trough? Nope. A simple way to get adequate calcium is by including the following foods in your diet: fortified grains, kale, collard greens, mustard greens, cabbage, kelp, seaweed, watercress, chickpeas, broccoli, red beans, soybeans, tofu, seeds (sesame seeds rate among the highest), and raw nuts. It is just that simple. But don't be looking to pop a calcium pill as a quick fix. Research shows that supplements do not make a significant difference in preventing or treating osteoporosis.[90] Good news: Fifteen minutes of direct sunlight every day aides in Vitamin D absorption, which means stronger bones.

How about eggs, you ask? When a woman is pregnant and she drinks alcohol or does drugs, it affects her unborn child, right? Right. Well, it is the same with chickens and their unhatched eggs. When you eat eggs, you are ingesting all the same hormones, pesticides, chemicals, and steroids as if you were eating the chicken directly. So if you really believe that eating "just egg whites" isn't fattening, we've got a bridge we can sell ya. Eggs are high in saturated fat and are completely disgusting when you think about what you are eating. Try that for once. Actually think about what you are eating!

You will pee in your pants when you see how much weight you lose from giving up dairy. The fat in cheese is what gives it the taste and texture we love. Of the calories found in cheese, 70 to 80 percent come from fat. Even if you're buying the low-fat, part-skim nonsense, more than half the calories come from fat.[91] Fat free?

Give us a freaking break! Remember what milk is for. It is designed to fatten up baby cows. Do you really believe it can be made fat free? Get your head out of your ass. Milk = fat. Butter = fat. Cheese = fat. People who think these products can be low fat or fat free = fucking morons.

Luckily, there are many alternatives to dairy products. Not only do grocery stores carry these items, but many coffee shops now offer soymilk and some bakeries are selling dairy-free desserts. A personal favorite-tasting milk substitute is Rice Dream (Original Enriched), which is fortified with vitamins and calcium. But feel free to experiment until you find your own favorite brand. Remember to read the ingredients. Avoid the milk substitutes that contain sugar. Instead of butter, try Earth Balance Natural Buttery Spread or Soy Garden Natural Buttery Spread, both made from nonhydrogenated oils. Can't live without ice cream? You don't have to. Soy Delicious has incredible knock-offs, which are completely dairy free. They even make must-have flavors, such as Chunky Mint Madness, Cookie Avalanche, Rocky Road, and Peanut Butter Zigzag. They also have a line of "ice creams" and sorbets that are fruit-sweetened! Dairy and sugar free! Too exciting for words! We're also huge fans of Double Rainbow Soy Cream, another amazing ice cream alternative. Are you a cheese addict? No problem. Follow Your Heart's Vegan Gourmet makes a kick-ass substitute in mozzarella, Monterey jack, and nacho. It even melts! It rules. Beware of the many brands that tout themselves as "soy cheese," leading consumers to believe they're dairy free. When you get past the misleading packaging and actually read the ingredients, you'll discover sneaky dairy ingredients like whey or casein. Steer clear. Other brands are completely dairy-free, but they taste like shit.

Need eggs in your life? Easy peasy. Egg Beaters are made of real eggs, so they're a gross no-no. But if you pan-fry House Tofu Steak (slice it in half first) and add a little soy butter, salt, pepper, and ketchup, you've got yourself a fried "egg." There's also an egg substitute in powder form for cooking and baking called Ener-G egg replacer. And many markets sell a pretty good tofu "egg" salad.

As the demand grows for healthy, yummy, animal-free, dairy-free products, more companies will supply us with these foods. So let your consumer dollars voice your desire, and your body will be rewarded. And don't be shy. If your grocery store doesn't carry something you want, open your fat mouth and ask for it.

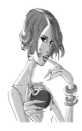

Chapter 6

You Are What You Eat

Now would be a good time to reflect on the old adage, "You are what you eat." This statement, in all its simplicity, is brilliant. You are what you eat. You are a human body comprised of organs, blood and guts, and other shit. The food you put into your body works its way through your organs and bloodstream and is actually part of who you are. So every time you put crap in your body, you are crap.

If Chapters 4 and 5 didn't convince you to avoid eating animal products (crap), maybe this will. Even knowing how abysmal the living conditions are for animals on factory farms, you cannot begin to imagine what the slaughter practices are like. "Humane" protocol calls for animals to be "stunned" before they are slaughtered. For cows, this means getting a metal bolt shot into the skull and then retracted. When done properly, using working equipment, this renders the cow unconscious. But time is money, and slaughterhouses operate at lightning speeds, some killing one animal every three seconds. Because thousands of frightened, struggling cows are not easy to stun, it is extremely common for a "stunner" to miss his mark.[92] Panicked hogs, also difficult to "hit," are stunned with an electric device. And if the jolt is too high, it bruises and bloodies the hogs' flesh (bad for business). Because business comes first on factory farms, the jolt is lowered, despite the fact that it doesn't properly stun the hogs.[93]

Stunned or not, cows and hogs are then "strung up" from the ceiling by a chain attached to their leg(s).[94] In theory, while they dangle there, they are supposed to be unconscious. But often they are fully conscious, struggling, screaming, and fearfully staring at the workers while they have their throats stabbed open.[95] Next, they travel along a "bleed rail," where they should bleed to death. But again, these large, frightened, struggling, conscious animals are difficult targets and the "stickers" (workers who cut their throats) don't always get a "good cut." Before cows can bleed to death, they are sent on their way to the "head-skinners," where the skin is sliced from their heads while they are still conscious.[96] Of course, this is excruciatingly painful, and the cows kick and struggle frantically. To avoid getting injured by the struggling animal, workers will sometimes sever the spinal cord with a knife blow to the back of the head. This paralyzes the animal below the neck so that the worker is safe. But these cows can still feel their skin being sliced away from their faces.[97] Next, their legs and head are chopped off, their entrails removed from their bodies, and then, finally, they are split in half. Often before hogs can bleed to death, they are dunked fully conscious into 140-degree scalding water to remove the hair from their bodies.[98]

Chickens, because they are so overcrowded and stressed, frequently peck each other and factory farm workers, so the ends of their beaks are literally chopped off their faces. Even though they currently comprise more than 95 percent of all animals slaughtered for food, Congress exempted chickens (and turkeys) from the Humane Slaughter Act, so there is no requirement to stun them[99] (not that it would matter, anyway). But because it is easier to handle chickens that aren't fighting for their lives, their heads are sometimes dragged through a water bath that has been electrically charged. This paralyzes the birds, but does not render them unconscious.[100] They are snatched up, shackled upside down, and their throats are slashed by machine at the rate of thousands per hour.[101] Next, they are dunked in scalding water to loosen their feathers. Again, they are supposed to be dead at this point, but if the machine misses its mark, or the chickens haven't bled to death, they are "boiled" alive. Then they are placed into a series of machines that literally beat their feathers off of them, still alive and having just been scalded.[102] All the while, they are being handled like rubber toys: grabbed by their necks, feet, or wings and thrown around. You get the idea.

In egg-laying factories, male baby chicks are completely useless to farmers because they don't produce eggs. So workers snatch up chicks speeding by on a conveyer belt, quickly glance at their undersides, and then toss the "useless" males into the garbage. Yes. Literally. Millions of male baby chicks are piled on top of each other in garbage dumpsters—left to die.

In her book, *Slaughterhouse,* Gail Eisnitz, chief investigator for the Humane Farming Association, interviewed dozens of slaughter-house workers throughout the country. *Every single one* admitted to abusing animals or neglecting to report those who did.[103] The following are quotes from slaughterhouse workers taken from her book. (They are quite graphic and difficult to read, but we implore you to read each one. It is important to know what our dietary desires are contributing to. Surely you can endure reading it if animals have to endure suffering it):

"I seen them take those stunners—they're about as long as a yard stick—and shove it up the hog's ass. . . They do it with cows, too. . . And in their ears, their eyes, down their throat. . . They'll be squealing and they'll just shove it right down there."[104]

"Hogs get stressed out pretty easy. If you prod them too much they have heart attacks. If you get a hog in a chute that's had the shit prodded out of him and has a heart attack or refuses to move, you take a meat hook and hook it into his bunghole [anus]. You're dragging these hogs alive, and a lot of times the meat hook rips out of the bunghole. I've seen hams—thighs—completely ripped open. I've also seen intestines come out. If the hog collapses near the front of the chute, you shove the meat hook into his cheek and drag him forward."[105]

"Or in their mouth. The roof of their mouth. And they're still alive."[106]

"Pigs on the kill floor have come up and nuzzled me like a puppy. Two minutes later I had to kill them—beat them to death with a pipe."[107]

"These hogs get up to the scalding tank, hit the water and start screaming and kicking. Sometimes they thrash so much they kick water out of the tank. . . . Sooner or later they drown. There's a rotating arm that pushes them under, no chance for them to get out. I'm not sure if they burn to death before they drown, but it takes them a couple of minutes to stop thrashing."[108]

"Sometimes I grab it [a hog] by the ear and stick it right through the eye. I'm not just taking its eye out, I'll go all the way to the hilt, right up through the brain, and wiggle the knife."[109]

"Only you don't just kill it, you go in hard, push hard, blow the windpipe, make it drown in its own blood. Split its nose. A live hog would be running around the pit. It would just be looking up at me and I'd be sticking, and I would just take my knife and—cut its eye out while it was just sitting there. And this hog would just scream."[110]

"I could tell you horror stories . . . about cattle getting their heads stuck under the gate guards, and the only way you can get it out is to cut their heads off while they're still alive."[111]

"He'll kick them [hogs], fork them, use anything he can get his hands on. He's already broken three pitchforks so far this year, just jabbing them. He doesn't care if he hits its eyes, head, butt. He jabs them so hard he busts the wooden handles. And he clubs them over the back."[112]

"I've seen live animals shackled, hoisted, stuck, and skinned. Too many to count, too many to remember. It's just a process that's continually there. I've seen shackled beef looking around before they've been stuck. I've seen hogs [that are supposed to be lying down] on the bleeding conveyor get up after they've been stuck. I've seen hogs in the scalding tub trying to swim."[113]

"I seen guys take broomsticks and stick it up the cow's behind, screwing them with a broom."[114]

"I've drug cows till their bones start breaking, while they were still alive. Bringing them around the corner and they get stuck up in the doorway, just pull them till their hide be ripped, till the blood just drip on the steel and concrete. Breaking their legs. . . . And the cow be crying with its tongue stuck out. They pull him till his neck just pop."[115]

"One time I took my knife—it's sharp enough—and I sliced off the end of a hog's nose, just like a piece of bologna. The hog went crazy for a few seconds. Then it just sat there looking kind of stupid. So I took a handful of salt brine and ground it into his nose. Now that hog really went nuts, pushing its nose all over the place. I still had a bunch of salt left in my hand—I was wearing a rubber glove—and I stuck the salt right up the hog's ass. The poor hog didn't know whether to shit or go blind."[116]

"Nobody knows who's responsible for correcting animal abuse at the plant. The USDA does zilch."[117]

Eisnitz chronicled the constant failure of U.S. Department of Agriculture inspectors to stop this abuse and their willingness to look the other way. In addition, she exposed the USDA's blatant tolerance for allowing contaminated meat into the human food supply. Think about it. *Ten billion* animals a year! Do you think the USDA has enough inspectors to supervise the humane and safe slaughter of *10 billion* animals a year? Of course the inspectors tolerate abuse and contaminated meat. Imagine the kind of person who would have a job that entailed witnessing the slaughter of thousands of innocent animals every day. Even if every single inspector did a good job (they don't), the factory workers can easily bypass the system. Eisnitz interviewed one worker from a horse slaughterhouse, who said, "Might be part of him's [a contaminated horse] bad, might be the pneumonia's traveled everywhere. I'd drag him back, and my boss would tell me to cut the hindquarters off and bring him into the cooler. The meat's supposed to be condemned, but still you'd cut it up and bag it." When Eisnitz asked, "But don't they have to be stamped 'USDA inspected?' " he responded, "He [his boss] got the stamper. He can stamp it himself when the doc leaves. . . . You take a condemned horse, skin him, cut him up, sell the meat. . . . We've sold it as beef."[118]

According to the Congressional testimony of one former Perdue worker, the poultry plants are filthy. She said there were flies, rats, and 5-inch long flying cockroaches covering the walls and floors.[119] Believe it or not, it gets worse: "After they are hung, sometimes the chickens fall off into the drain that runs down the middle of the line. This is where roaches, intestines, diseased parts, fecal contamination, and blood are washed down. Workers [vomit] into the drain. . . . Employees are constantly chewing and spitting out snuff and tobacco on the floor . . . sometimes they have to relieve themselves on the floor. . . . The Perdue supervisors told us to take the fallen chickens out of the drain and send them down the line."[120] A USDA inspector said of the cockroaches, "One time we shined a flashlight into a hole they were crawling in and out, and they were so thick it was like maggots, you couldn't even see the surface."[121] A worker at another poultry plant said, "Every day, I saw black chicken, green chicken, chicken that stank, and chicken with feces on it. Chicken like this is supposed to be thrown away, but instead it would be sent down the line to be processed."[122] Another worker at another plant said, "I personally have seen rotten meat—you can tell by the odor. This rotten meat is mixed with the fresh meat and sold for baby food. We are asked to mix it with the fresh food, and this is the way it is sold. You can see the worms inside the meat."[123] No comment. We are simply speechless.

Animals are intelligent, emotional, social creatures. Researchers at Bristol University in Britain discovered that cows actually nurture friendships and bear grudges. One study showed cows displaying excitement while solving intellectual challenges.[124]

Chickens are as smart as mammals, including some primates,

claims animal behaviorist Dr. Chris Evans of Macquarie University in Australia. They are apt pupils and can learn by watching the mistakes of others. One researcher conducted a study that demonstrated chickens' ability to use switches and levers to change the temperature of their surroundings. A PBS documentary revealed chickens' love for television and music.[125]

Pigs can play video games! They've been labeled as more intelligent than dogs and three-year-old humans. They too can indicate their temperature preferences.[126]

Even fish have feelings. Dr. Donald Broom, scientific adviser to the British government, explains, "The scientific literature is quite clear. Anatomically, physiologically and biologically, the pain system in fish is virtually the same as in birds and animals." Fish, like "higher vertebrates," have neurotransmitters similar to endorphins that relieve suffering. Of course, the only reason for their nervous systems to produce painkillers is to relieve pain.[127]

Animals hear the screaming and crying of other animals being slaughtered and are terrified. They know they are about to be killed and they are panic-stricken. When their young are taken from them, cows kick stall walls in rage and frustration and literally cry with grief.

Think of how you feel when you are angry, afraid, and grief-stricken. Bear in mind the physical feelings that accompany these emotions. These emotions—fear, grief, and rage—produce chemical changes in our bodies. They do the same to animals. Their blood pressures rise. Adrenaline courses through their bodies. You are eating high blood pressure, stress, and adrenaline. You are eating fear, grief, and rage. You are eating suffering, horror, and murder. You are eating cruelty. You are what you eat. You cannot be thin and beautiful with a glowing complexion when you eat fear, grief, and rage.

Although a minuscule percentage of "meat" in the United States comes from free-range farms, how do you even know it is really free-range? Companies want us to believe that products labeled "free-range" or "free-roaming" are derived from animals that spent their short lives outdoors, enjoying sunshine, fresh air, and the company of other animals. But labels—other than "organic" on egg cartons—are not subject to any government regulations. In addition, the USDA doesn't regulate "free-range" or "free-roaming" claims for beef products.[128] Because there are no agencies governing these claims, do you take the word of someone who makes a living on blood money? And even if the farm was free-range and humane, the animals are still being sent to horrific slaughterhouses. (An undercover video of a kosher slaughterhouse revealed animals suffering the same abuse and torture.)[129] Many animals don't even survive the transport from their factory or free-range farm to slaughter. The only law in existence dictating care for transported animals is related to *train* transport. But it just so happens that 95 percent of animals are transported by *truck*.[130] They receive no food or water and no protection from the elements. Hundreds of thousands of animals are dead on arrival or too injured or sick to move. They don't get to stop for bathroom breaks, so the animals are forced to stand in their own urine and feces. In the wintertime, the animals' flesh and feet will actually freeze to the bottom and sides of the truck. So upon arrival, they are literally ripped away from the truck. One worker interviewed by Eisnitz said, "They freeze to that steel railing. They're still alive, and they'll hook a cable on it and pull it out, maybe pull a leg off."[131]

Assuming you started with a healthy animal (highly unlikely), you've now eaten hormones, pesticides, steroids, antibiotics, fear, grief, and rage. You are what you eat. But what if the animal wasn't healthy? Animals that are too sick or injured to walk are literally dragged to slaughter, one end of a chain attached to the animal, the other to a truck. The USDA still allowed these animals, referred to as "downers," to be slaughtered for human consumption until 2004. Finally, with the outbreak of more mad cow disease cases (a deadly and incurable disease that can be transmitted to humans through the consumption of cow flesh), they came to their senses. But in 2005, USDA Secretary Mike Johanns announced that downed animals may once again be slaughtered for human food. So in addition to all the other filth you're eating, you're also eating whatever illness the animal had. You are what you eat.

Let's make believe that all the animals killed for human consumption are healthy, happy, free of antibiotics, steroids, and pesticides and are humanely raised and slaughtered. Pretend you are eating "perfect meat." Great. But what exactly are you eating? "Meat" is the decomposing, decaying, rotting flesh of a dead animal. As soon as an animal dies, it starts "breaking down." How long has passed between when the animal was slaughtered and the time you are eating it? It could be weeks, even months. You want to put a dead animal corpse—that has been rotting away for months—in your mouth? In your body? Because meat is muscle tissue, it oxidizes in an open environment and turns brown. So most meat markets will scrape off the brown parts to make it look more appealing. Another trick of the trade is using tinted lighting in open meat cases to enhance the meat's color.[132] Restaurants and ranchers might call their meat "aged to perfection," but no matter how you slice it, it's still a putrefying corpse. You are what you eat.

Just because you can't see what's happening doesn't mean it doesn't exist. Every time you have a craving for meat or dairy, remember what goes on inside every slaughterhouse, processing plant, and grocery store. Linda McCartney said it best: "If slaughterhouses had glass walls, we'd all be vegetarians."[133] For added motivation with your new lifestyle, visit GoVeg.com and order a free vegetarian starter kit.

So now you are officially vegan, a person who doesn't eat *any* animal products. No meat, chicken, pork, fish, eggs, milk, cheese, or butter. Feel great about it. Yes, it is challenging to avoid these foods, but you will reap the karmic rewards of being vegan (like being skinny). For starters, you're sparing the lives of at least ninety animals a year.[134] And every environmentalist knows that factory farming is completely destroying the environment. As ridiculous as it sounds, the methane resulting from the burps and farts of 10 billion animals a year is directly responsible for global warming.[135] The urine and feces are polluting and contaminating soil and water all over the country. According to the Environmental Protection Agency, they are the largest polluters of U.S. waterways.[136] Moreover, the amount of land, food, water, and energy used to raise 10 billion animals a year for slaughter could be used to grow food for *all of the starving people in the world.* That's right—you being vegan is actually a step toward ending world hunger. Now that's some serious skinny karma.

So you shouldn't eat cows, chickens, pigs, fish, milk, cheese, or eggs. So what the hell should you eat? Pretty much everything else: fruits, vegetables, legumes, nuts, seeds, and whole grains. Deep down, you've known all along that these foods are best for you; now it's time to get back on track. Our diets have strayed so far off course from where they belong; we've allowed meat to take center stage, with grains and vegetables playing supporting roles. Wrong, wrong, wrong. There is a plethora of great-tasting, healthy, wholesome foods that you've likely been neglecting for years. Well, those days are over.

Can you remember back to your grade-school days when you

learned about photosynthesis? Plants store the sun's energy, which we receive by eating them. If you can, just picture the light energy from the sun beaming down to the vegetables and fruits, and as we eat those foods, imagine that energy being transmitted into our bodies. Our nervous systems are maintained and stimulated by this light. What an amazing gift from nature—to be able to eat such pure foods that give our bodies so much!

However, be advised, all fruits and vegetables are not created equal. Plants need vitamins and minerals to function and grow properly. When they are sprayed with pesticides and grown in chemically treated soil, they won't absorb all the proper nutrients. This results in a loss of enzymes. So, organic fruits and vegetables— ones that have been grown in pure, untreated soil and without pesticides—have far more enzymes than their conventionally grown counterparts.[137]

Any scientist can tell you that food has an "energy" or "life" to it. Anyone with common sense can tell you that eating a live, fresh fruit is healthier than eating a cooked, canned, preserved one. Why? Because this "life" comes from the plant's energy, nutrients, phytochemicals, and enzymes. Enzymes are living biochemical fac-

tors that we need to survive. They are critical for digestion, breathing, reproduction, and the functioning of DNA and RNA. They
also help repair and heal our organs, detoxify our bodies, carry out
our nerve impulses, and help us think.

There are three types of enzymes: metabolic, digestive, and food
enzymes. Fortunately, we produce our own metabolic enzymes,
which run the whole body, maintain our health, and defend us from
illness and infection. But our own enzyme supplies are limited. So
to continue healthy bodily functions, we need to supplement with
food. When we eat, our bodies release digestive enzymes to break
down the food. If we eat foods devoid of enzymes, such as meat,
processed food, and even just overcooked food (high temperatures
destroy enzymes), our bodies have to work much harder.[138] Harder
work means using more of our precious enzymes. Over time, this
can result in an enlargement of the digestive organs and the
endocrine glands. (Studies have shown that the increased weight of
these organs accompanies obesity.)[139] This lack of enzymes can also
cause a disruption in the body's ability to make enough metabolic
enzymes. But when we eat foods high in enzymes, such as fruits,
salad, or lightly steamed veggies, we get an enzyme boost along

with the meal, so our bodies don't have to work so hard. There is no greater defender of our bodies than enzymes. When not in use for digestion, enzymes are busy repairing and cleaning our bodies.[140] So don't go throwing your enzymes away on shit!

So how do we get these enzymes into our bodies? We just need to make the following foods part of our daily diets: fruits (especially pineapples, papayas, bananas, and mangos), raw or lightly steamed vegetables, raw nuts and seeds, wheat grass, sea vegetables, garlic, and legumes. Juicing is a great way to detoxify your body and get a lot of enzymes, but you must drink it right away.[141] As soon as a fruit is peeled, or cut, or juiced, it begins to lose its enzymes.[142] So, buying a gallon of fresh-squeezed juice isn't as beneficial as making your own daily. Packaged juice has been pasteurized, and the heat destroys the enzymes. Granted, it's still better to drink pasteurized juice than soda. So if you can't juice for yourself, do the best you can.

Well, there you have it. Fruits and vegetables are the answer. And unless you are an idiot who wants cancer, obesity, and enlarged organs, organic is the way to go. You are what you eat.

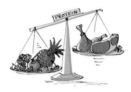

Chapter 7

The Myths and Lies About Protein

If we had a penny for every time some meathead asked us, "So where do you get your protein?" we'd be richer than Oprah. Have you ever, ever, ever, in your entire life, heard of anyone suffering from a protein deficiency? Did you ever see an elephant, moose, or giraffe jonesing for a protein fix? If you weren't blacked out on bourbon for the past three chapters, you should

know by now: It is a complete myth that we need a massive amount
of protein. Too much protein—especially animal protein—can
impair our kidneys; leach calcium, zinc, vitamin B, iron, and magnesium from our bodies; and cause osteoporosis, heart disease, cancer,
and obesity. In addition, high amounts of protein can damage our
tissues, organs, and cells, contributing to faster aging.[143] Yikes!
Know this: People in other cultures consume half the amount of
protein that we do, yet they live longer, healthier lives.[144]

Although too much is harmful, protein is still vital to our health.
Protein produces enzymes, hormones, neurotransmitters, and anti-
bodies; replaces worn out cells; transports various substances
throughout the body; and aids in growth and repair.[145]

So how much protein do we really need? Well, depending who
you ask, that number varies anywhere from 18 to 60 grams a day.
But one thing is certain: Vegetarians need not worry. Researchers
at Harvard found that vegetarians (who don't live on junk food) get
adequate amounts of protein in their diets.[146] The American
Dietetic Association reports that eating a vegetarian diet provides
twice the amount of protein needed daily.[147] In his book, *Optimal
Health,* Dr. Patrick Holford explains that "most people are in more

danger of eating too much protein than too little."[148] So pick something else to be neurotic about.

How do vegans get protein? Simply. We eat lentils, beans, nuts,
seeds, fruits, vegetables, whole grains, and soy products (edamame,
tofu, imitation cheeses and meats). When you eat well-balanced
meals consisting of these foods, you are guaranteed to get sufficient
protein. For example, for lunch, if you had a soy burger on a whole
grain bun with avocado and tomato and a small side salad, you'd get
22 grams of protein. See how easy? If you want an extra boost, treat
yourself to spirulina, a high-protein algae that contains omega-3
and omega-6 fatty acids, B-12 (important for vegetarians),
enzymes, and minerals. It also supports the immune system, fights
cancer, and helps with hypoglycemia, anemia, ulcers, diabetes, and
chronic fatigue syndrome. Spirulina also contains all nine essential
amino acids.[149]

Amino acids, huh? Yep. There are twenty amino acids. Our bodies produce eleven, and the other nine essential amino acids can be
obtained through food. Amino acids are the building blocks of protein. And yes, protein does build muscle. But even if you work out
and want to build muscle, you don't need to overdose on animal

protein (a ridiculous myth perpetuated by the health club industry). Bear in mind, some top athletes are vegetarians: Chris Campbell is an Olympic wrestling champion; Keith Holmes, a world-champion middleweight boxer; Bill Mannetti, a power-lifting champion; Bill Pearl, a four-time Mr. Universe; Andres Cahling, a champion body-builder and Olympic gold medalist in the ski jump; Art Still, a Hall of Famer and MVP defensive end for the NFL; Martina Navratilova, a tennis champion; and Dr. Ruth Heidrich, a six-time Ironwoman, age-group record holder, USA track and field Master's Champion, and vegan.[150]

Another common myth that has since been debunked is the "food combining" theory. Animal flesh proteins are "complete," meaning they contain all nine essential amino acids in amounts similar to those found in human flesh. Plants have all these amino acids, too, just in slightly different amounts. It was previously believed that in order to create complete proteins from vegetarian foods, you needed to combine them in specific ways. For example, it was said rice and beans had to be eaten together to maximize their protein potential. However, it is now known that eating a variety of foods from plant sources provides all the building blocks we need. Further, the microorganisms and recycled cells in our intestinal tracts make complete proteins for us.[151] All we have to do is eat healthy, balanced diets.

An integral part of any healthy, balanced diet is fat. Don't cringe. Fat doesn't always mean fattening. Essential fatty acids provide us with energy and offer protection from heart disease, stroke, and high blood pressure. They also combat allergies, premenstrual syndrome, arthritis, and skin problems.[152] Our brilliant bodies make all the essential fatty acids we need, except for two: linoleic and linolenic acids, also known as omega-3 and omega-6.[153] These *good fats* are found in olive oil, sesame oil, canola oil, flaxseed oil, hempseed oil, evening primrose oil, raw nuts and seeds, and avocados. So quit listening to all the stupid bitches who boycott nuts, oils, and avocados because they think they're fattening. Even though they're high in fat, they will not make you fat (unless you totally overdose on them). Unsaturated fats such as these are good for your body, and when eaten as part of a well-balanced vegan diet, they don't make you fat! It's the saturated fats, found in meat, dairy, and hydrogenated oils that make you fat. Think about the source of the oils or fats and use your head. Do you think an avocado, which is a fruit, is going to turn you into a hippo? Common sense, bitches.

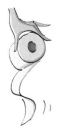

Chapter 8

Pooping

P inch a loaf. Lay cable. Drop the kids off at the pool. Let's face it; there is no greater pleasure than taking a big, steamy dump. But shitting isn't just for kicks. It is a vital tool for weight loss and optimal health. Basic math, girls. How much are you putting in your mouth, and how much is coming out your ass? Now that you've learned the right foods to eat and which ones to avoid, you should be a dynamo in the bathroom. But if your hiney is only expelling little rabbit turds, something's gotta give.

Earlier, we mentioned that drinking lots of water helps rid your body of waste. We can't emphasize the importance of this enough. Drink, drink, drink. But if you want to take tyrannosaurus-sized dumps, it's also imperative to eat foods rich in fiber, like whole grain cereals and breads, brown rice, corn, barley, rye, buckwheat, millet, oats, fruits, vegetables (especially root vegetables, like carrots), beans, and seeds. Avoid foods that have little or no fiber, like meat, eggs, cheese, milk, and processed, refined foods. These can clog up your ass. (It is a myth that bananas are binding. Eat 'em.)

Fiber isn't just for shits and giggles, either. It offers protection from appendicitis, Candida, heart disease, high blood pressure, high cholesterol, diabetes, gallstones, irritable bowel syndrome (IBS), and colitis.[154] Fibrous foods also help normalize our blood-sugar levels, satiate food cravings, and make us feel fuller so that we don't overeat.[155] Fiber even fights colon and colorectal cancer, prostate cancer, and breast cancer: If we don't make ca-ca quickly enough, our putrefying food stays in our bodies, increasing the likelihood of the production of carcinogenic substances. [156] So eat your fiber, and crap like a champ.

Another way to get your bowels brewing is to pay special attention to the order in which you are eating foods. For example, foods that digest quickly and easily should be eaten by themselves and early in the day. Fruit for breakfast. Salad and/or vegetables for lunch. These foods will pass through your body at lightning speeds. Dinner should be your "heaviest" meal. Follow these simple rules and you'll be depositing six-inchers in no time. If you're already a quality dumper, feel free to disregard this paragraph.

But, if you still need an extra kick in the ass, up your bean intake. Beware: you might have a mudslide in your pants if you're not careful. If you're not accustomed to beans, ease in slowly and be sure you are near a toilet.

If your deuce-dropping still needs work, do not take laxatives. Yes, they make you poop, but they don't solve the underlying problem of why you're not pooping in the first place. Most laxatives are gastro-intestinal irritants—even the natural ones.[157] Stop looking for a quick fix. Just continue to drink a lot of water, exercise, and eat right, shitheads.

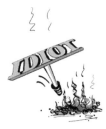

Chapter 9

Have No Faith: Governmental Agencies Don't Give a Shit About Your Health

The USDA: It's Not What You Think

President Abraham Lincoln founded the U.S. Department of Agriculture in 1862—when the majority of people were farmers and needed to exchange information about seeds and crops. In other words, the USDA was created to help farmers.

According to its web site, now, among other things, the USDA is responsible for "the safety of meat, poultry, and egg products."[158]

Hmm. That's weird. 'Cause many high-ranking staff members at the USDA were employed by, or are otherwise affiliated with, the meat and dairy industries.[159] And if the group responsible for "the safety of meat, poultry, and egg products" is run by people from the same industries they're supposed to be protecting us from . . . well, that would be a conflict of interest. *And it is.* An enormous, ridiculous, outrageous, catastrophic conflict of interest.

One former USDA Secretary was forced to resign amid charges of accepting illegal corporate gifts from seven different companies. He was indicted on thirty-nine felony counts, including tampering with a witness; accepting illegal gratuities; making false statements; and violating the Meat Inspection Act of 1907. (Tyson Foods, one of the companies that admitted to giving the Secretary corporate favors, was required to pay $4 million in fines and endure four years' probation. A mere slap on the wrist, when the USDA could've barred Tyson from selling food to military bases and schools. That would've really stung, considering Tyson sold more than $10 million worth of food to the Defense Department alone in 1996.[160] But friends don't treat each other that way.)

President George W. Bush's Agriculture Secretary from January 2001 until January 2005, Ann Veneman, not only had ties with the company responsible for producing the controversial bovine growth hormone, (BGH), but she was also linked to a major meatpacking corporation.[161] The buck doesn't stop there. She employed a spokeswoman who was the former public relations director for the Cattlemen's Beef Association, a chief of staff who used to be its head lobbyist, a former president of the National Pork Producers Council, and former executives from the meatpacking industry, just to name a few.[162]

Safety Last

With that in mind, it's no wonder Veneman vetoed a program that would test all U.S. cattle for mad cow disease. In fact, out of the 35 million cattle slaughtered in 2003, the USDA only tested 20,000 for mad cow disease. (Japan tests *all* of their cattle killed for human consumption.)[163] Of course it wouldn't be in a rancher's best interest to test all of his cattle. If they were inflicted with mad cow disease, he couldn't sell their meat, and he'd lose money. Heaven forbid the USDA risk a rancher's profits.

So, in order to appear somewhat concerned about the prevention of mad cow disease, the USDA often refers to an FDA ban, which prohibits the feeding of ground-up cattle meat to live cattle. Big whoop. Banning cannibalism is a no-brainer. But why even bother banning cannibalism when they still allow the feeding of *cattle blood* to young calves? Stanley Prusiner, a Nobel Prize Winner for his work on mad cow disease, refers to this practice as "a really stupid idea."[164] Think about it: A cow dies from mad cow disease, but no one knows, because it wasn't one of the .0005714% percent tested. Cattle ranchers are now forbidden to grind up this dead cow and feed it to other cows. But, they can give its blood to calves as part of their feed. How fucking stupid, disgusting, and dangerous is that?

The USDA also likes referring to another "safety" program in place, called The National Animal Identification System (NAIS). The NAIS is a system for identifying an animal's origin so that if its meat is found to be contaminated, it can be traced back to a specific farm. (Forget testing as a preventative measure. Implement a system for after someone eats contaminated meat and we need a recall.) Participation in this program is voluntary.[165] Wow, the USDA sure has tough rules governing the safety of our country's meat.

The USDA's web site describing the NAIS actually has a section on "confidentiality." It reads, "The NAIS will contain only information necessary for animal health officials to be able to track suspect animals and identify any other animals that may have been exposed to a disease. . . . To help assure participants that the information will be used only for animal health purposes, the information must be confidential. USDA and its State partners will work to protect data confidentiality."[166] What the fuck? The USDA will protect the data confidentiality of farms that are supplying the public with contaminated meat? Why don't they just give all the ranchers blowjobs, too?

Many savvy consumers are catching on, and they know they cannot trust the USDA. According to the Organic Consumers Association, "Lester Friedlander, a former USDA veterinarian, says he was told by USDA officials as far back as 1991 that if his testing ever found evidence of Mad Cow disease, he was to tell no one. He and other scientists say they know of cases where cows tested positive for the disease in laboratories but were ruled negative by the USDA."[167] Trust no one!

Illegal hormones are regularly pumped into veal calves, which are suspected of increasing the growth of cancer cells in the humans who eat them. The USDA has not only been accused of overlooking these practices, but also of falsifying lab results, altering records, and pressuring staff to lie about events.[168] Even the selfish whores who eat veal don't deserve that.

Business First

None of us deserved to be deceived all these years by the preposterous USDA Dietary Guidelines and Food Pyramid, either. In 1998, the Physicians Committee for Responsible Medicine (PCRM) filed a federal lawsuit against the USDA and the Department of Health and Human Services. PCRM claimed that federal laws were violated when the USDA selected six out of eleven people with financial ties to various food industries to serve on the Dietary Guidelines Advisory Committee. The committee members' affiliations included the American Meat Institute,

National Livestock and Beef Board, the American Egg Board, the National Dairy Promotion and Research Program, the National Dairy Council, Dannon Company (yogurt), Mead Johnson Nutritionals (milk-based infant formulas), Nestlé (milk-based formulas, ice cream, condensed milk), and Slim-Fast (milk-based diet products).[169] How dare they?

(On a sidenote, PCRM also charged that the Dietary Guidelines —which recommended dairy products—were racially biased, because most nonwhites are lactose-intolerant.[170] According to Johnson & Johnson, lactose intolerance affects "over 50 percent of the Hispanic American population, 75 percent of Native Americans, 80 percent of African Americans, and 90 percent of Asian Americans."[171] Why does Johnson & Johnson care about the millions of minorities suffering from lactose intolerance? Because they can target these individuals for buying Lactaid, a product they hawk for aiding in dairy digestion. Even though you are lactose intolerant and your body thoroughly rejects dairy products, eat them anyway. Just buy and take our drug so you don't feel sick afterwards. Ugh, that just makes us sick with rage.)

Got $19 billion? The milk industry does, so they've got the USDA in their back pocket.[172] The California Milk Processor Board

(CMPB) was established in 1993 to increase milk sales in California. They were responsible for the campaigns that targeted children: "Got milk?" and "Milk. It does a body good." The CMPB is funded by all California milk processors, but administered by the California Department of Food and Agriculture. The National Fluid Milk Processor Promotion Board (Fluid Board) conceived of the "Milk Mustache" campaign, which targets young adults. The USDA's Agriculture Monitoring Service administers the Fluid Board.[173] Meaning, in essence, the California Department of Agriculture and the USDA are managing advertising campaigns for the milk industry. Under the guise of advancing health, they managed to dupe President Bill Clinton, while he was in office, into posing for their ads. They also had the audacity to feature the Secretary of Health and Human Services, Donna Shalala, sporting that stupid "milk mustache."[174] The Secretary of Health and Human Services using her status and title to promote a commercial product! Would she appear in ads for Pepsi or Nike? Say it out loud: conflict of interest. They've even got the U.S. surgeon general in on the act. In the first-ever report on "the state of the nation's bones," the U.S. surgeon general warned of an impending "osteoporosis crisis" expected by

the year 2020. In order to ward off this potential disaster, the
Surgeon General's report recommended three glasses of milk a day.
Guess who issued the report? The Department of Health and
Human Services.[175] Trust no one.

The horrors committed by the USDA could fill an entire book.
But we shouldn't be surprised. Although they don't list it as part of
their primary mission statement, the USDA does admit to being
"committed to helping America's farmers and ranchers."[176] The
same USDA responsible for "the safety" of meat, poultry, dairy,
and eggs also promotes the sale of them. In fact, they even go so far
as to purchase the products themselves, using *our* tax dollars. The
USDA will spend $30 million a year on beef buyouts alone.
Another $30 million of *our* hard-earned money goes toward pork
purchases.[177] Wow. It must be nice for these industries to have the
USDA bailing them out whenever they have a surplus of items.
What, exactly, do they do with all this food that *we* pay for?

All in a Day's Work

Ever hear of the National School Lunch Program (NSLP)? It's
a nation-wide $4 billion scheme that allows the USDA to buy

up all this meat, milk, and cheese with our tax dollars, and then dump this crap into the bodies of more than 26 million school children.[178] Ever wonder why school lunches are *required* to include milk? The NSLP directly benefits the meat, dairy, and poultry industries at the expense of our nation's children.

In 1999, a ground beef plant in Texas failed a series of USDA tests for salmonella. The tests showed that as much as 47 percent of the company's ground beef contained salmonella—a proportion 5 times higher than what USDA regulations allow. Despite this, and the fact that high levels of salmonella in ground beef indicate high levels of fecal contamination, the USDA continued to purchase thousands of tons of the meat for distribution in schools. In fact, this company was one of the nation's largest suppliers for the school meals, providing as much as 45 percent of the program's ground meat.[179]

Contamination aside, according to Michele Simon of the Center for Informed Food Choices, "One evaluation of the commodity foods program estimates that 70 percent of the items offered exceed the U.S. dietary guidelines for fat."[180] For decades, consumer advocacy groups have been horrified by this unhealthy, profit-driven arrangement. With the backing of countless parents, physicians, and nutritionists, they have battled to get soy milk and other healthier choices approved by the USDA for use in school lunches. But the USDA (a.k.a.: the beef, pork, poultry, and dairy industries) wants no part in this, of course.

The USDA has fifteen food-assistance programs, including ones for the elderly, homeless, military, and poor. It is estimated that one in five Americans will take part in this $41.6 billion program.[181] Sounds like the USDA is helping to feed a lot of people, right? Right. They are feeding them fattening, unhealthy, artery-clogging, heart-stopping, acid-producing, contaminated meat, poultry, and dairy—with our money. How generous.

Organic or Not?

It's not enough that they dictate all things meat and dairy, the USDA even sticks its big nose into our organic products, too. In April 2004, the USDA made sweeping changes to their National Organic Program (NOP) standards. The new rules infuriated organic farmers and consumers because: Livestock were allowed to eat non-organic fishmeal, even if it contained toxins or synthetic preservatives; cows and calves given growth hormones, antibiotics, or other drugs could still provide the public with "organic" milk, as long as a year had passed since the drugs were administered; pesticides could be used even if they contained unknown inert ingredients as long as a "reasonable effort" had been made to identify them; and seafood, pet food, clothing, fertilizers, and body care products could be labeled organic without being monitored by the USDA.[183] Not only were people livid with the actual changes, but also with the decision-making process. By law, these types of regulatory changes are required to undergo a period of public comment before being enacted. There was no comment period, just an announcement of changes after the fact.[184]

According to Ronnie Cummins, national director of Organic Consumers Association (OCA), "Rather than comply with regulations which uphold the integrity of organic food, corporate-run factory farms, who want a piece of the $11 billion a year organic industry, are manipulating the USDA and Congress to change the rules to suit their toxic-industrial style of farming. Allowing non-organic, and potentially genetically engineered feed to be included under the definition of "organic" is a major setback for the integrity of what is the fastest-growing sector of the food industry in this country."[185] Thanks to the phone calls, letters, e-mails, and faxes of many pissed off consumers, the USDA reversed all these changes in May 2004.[186]

Even so, many people are still mistrustful of the USDA. Nonprofit group, The Center for Food Safety (CFS), claims that the USDA may be allowing "sham" certifiers under the umbrella of the National Organic Program (NOP). Their suspicions were aroused by the high volume of certifications issued within a short time. These worries were heightened when the USDA refused to provide CFS with requested documents, even though they were required to do so under the Freedom of Information Act.[187]

Other environmental groups along with the OCA have joined a lawsuit against the USDA. Among their complaints was the fact that the USDA's NOP created an additional category of certified products, which directly opposes legislation put in place by Congress. They state, "When Congress has spoken clearly on a sub-ject, USDA has no discretion to rewrite the statute making exceptions that dilute the standards of the Act."[188] Can you believe the nerve of these USDA fuckers? Going against laws created by our elected officials and making up their own rules? It's fucking mutiny, is what it is. Trust no one.

When buying organic foods, look for certification from anyone other than the USDA. Oregon Tilth, California Certified Organic Farmers, Marin Organic Certifying Agency, and Demeter Certified Biodynamic are all reputable. Sometimes a product will be certified organic by the USDA and another party. So don't rule it out just because the USDA certifies it.

Surely you've seen the "organic" Horizon brand of dairy products in your grocery store? It is the nation's largest supplier of organic dairy products. Well, it just so happens that Horizon has been accused of violating organic standards. The Cornucopia Institute, a watchdog group in support of organic agriculture, filed two complaints with the USDA. They allege that two major farms that supply Horizon with milk are confining cows in an industrial setting and denying them access to pasture, yet are still calling their products organic.[189]

Why is all this allowed to happen? Don't our elected officials know what's going on? Why don't they try to stop this? Some do. But many politicians are in bed with the evil industries. McDonald's alone has made close to $2 million in campaign contributions; the National Cattlemen's Beef Association nearly $1.5 million; and the National Restaurant Association more than $3.1 million.[190] Hate to sound like a broken record player, but trust no one.

Is Everyone in the FDA on Drugs?

This greed-induced immorality isn't applicable just to Congress or the USDA. The Food and Drug Administration (FDA) is a pathetic facade, too. In 1990, the Monsanto Company sought FDA approval for Posilac, a commercialized form of bovine growth hormone (BGH, used to increase cows' milk production). Even though the test study linked the hormone to prostate and thyroid cancer, the FDA still approved Posilac. Of course, these damning test results weren't made available to the public until 1998, when a group of scientists conducted an independent analysis of the study. They found that the FDA never even reviewed Monsanto's findings! More recently, BGH has been linked to increased levels of Insulin Growth Factor-1, a cancer promoter. But the FDA has no interest in these findings, either. Or the fact that both the World Trade Organization and The United Nations Food Standards Body refuse to endorse the hormone's safety. And they certainly don't mind that BGH milk is banned in all of the European Union, Canada, Japan, and every other industrialized country in the world.[191] Fucking Dumb Asses.

Why would the FDA knowingly allow a cancer-causing hormone into our milk supply? One theory highlights the fact that the FDA Deputy Commissioner at the time of the Posilac approval was a former Monsanto lawyer. And, during his tenure at the FDA, this same deputy commissioner wrote the policy exempting BGH from special labeling. Yet, fingers also point to a former top scientist with Monsanto, who was hired by the FDA to review her *own* research, conducted while she was working for Monsanto. This little beauty also allowed a hundred-fold increase of antibiotic residues in milk.[192]

Fear not. The FDA's bad behavior isn't singular to the dairy industry. It also has a sketchy history with monosodium glutamate (MSG). One former FDA Commissioner testified before the Senate Select Committee on Nutrition that MSG was safe, citing four sources. It was later discovered that two of the studies were nonexistent, and the other two were incomplete![193]

Secrets and lies. It's just too much to bear. So let's also play the "I'm not telling" game. Ever see the words "natural flavors" on food packaging ingredient lists? Yeah, that's because the FDA allows companies to be vague and doesn't require them to tell us exactly what we're eating. The FDA has a list of approximately 300 foods that meet a "standard of identity," meaning, companies aren't required to spell out their ingredients. For example, ice cream manufacturers can use any of twenty-five specified additives without listing them in their ingredients.[194] Who wants to put something into his or her body without even knowing what it is? By now, Chapter 9, *you* better fucking not!

You Are Your Only Chance

If you want to get skinny, you can only rely on yourself. If you adapt only one practice from this book, let it be this: *Read the ingredients.* Forget counting carbs, adding calories, and multiplying fat grams. Just read the ingredients. It doesn't matter how many calories or carbs or fat grams something has. *It just doesn't matter.* You don't need the government's asinine recommended daily allowances (RDA) to tell you how to eat. Just read the ingredients. If they are healthy, wholesome, and pure—dive in. If there is refined sugar, white or bleached flour, hydrogenated oils, any animal products, artificial anything, or some scary-looking word that you don't know—don't eat it. We can't make it any simpler. Just read the ingredients and completely ignore all the other gibber jabber bullshit the government calls for on the packaging. Fuck them. Trust no one. Get skinny.

And no matter what, do not fall prey to clever advertising used on the packaging. The companies that call their products "wholesome" or "nutritious" can be the same ones that add hydrogenated oils, artificial flavors, or synthetic preservatives. Just read the ingredients of everything you buy. It's not a big deal, assuming you are literate.

There is so much bureaucracy and red tape surrounding health-related government agencies that you are much better off fending for yourself. After all, why would anyone take nutritional advice from organizations that let color dyes, hydrogenated oils, chemical preservatives, and artificial flavors into the food we eat?

The EPA Makes Us Sick

StarLink corn, a genetically modified organism, contains an insecticidal protein, deemed unsafe for human consumption. But the Environmental Protection Agency allows the use of StarLink for livestock feed.[195] Let humans eat the animals who ate the corn? That's safe? Duh.

Clearly, nothing is sacred to the group that allows *rocket fuel* in our milk supply. Yeah, you heard right. Rocket fuel. In milk. Thanks to the Pentagon, ammonium perchlorate, the main explosive component in rocket fuel, has been lurking around our environment for decades. It finds its way into water used for growing feed crops for cattle. Cows eat these contaminated crops, with the result being contaminated milk. Whether you are drinking milk or eating dairy products made with this milk, you are ingesting perchlorate. And the EPA actually makes allowances for a "provisional daily safe dose."[196] We're sorry, but where we're from—Earth—there is no acceptable amount to ingest where explosive components are concerned. Even if you believe any amount to be safe, tests revealed milk perchlorate levels well above the EPA's index. Studies conducted by the Environmental Working Group (EWG), a nonprofit, non-partisan organization, found *every single* milk sample tested in Texas to be contaminated. California's own Food and Agriculture Department found that milk off the grocers' shelves had *five times* the EPA's "safe dose" of perchlorate. But, of course, the California Food and Agriculture Department did not release these results. Instead, they were brought to light by the EWG. Although both the dairy industry and government agencies acknowledge that there could be some health risks associated with perchlorate, they maintain that we should keep drinking milk for its "calcium, protein and minerals."[197] We'll let you use your own heads on this one.

Regardless of your political affiliation, please know this: The Bush Administration continuously asks for exemptions on behalf of the military and chemical companies, allowing them to continue this contamination and to shirk responsibility for cleanup. In fact, the Bush administration's EPA has been widely criticized on many counts of environmental pollution that affect our food and water supply. Like the USDA's pathetic voluntary program, the EPA has its own version of letting agribusiness trample all over public health and safety. Collaborating closely with the U.S. Poultry and Egg Association and

The National Pork Producers Council (NPPC), the EPA developed a *voluntary* air-monitoring program. Disregard the notion that the EPA blames factory farming for 73 percent of all ammonia (fumes from all the shit and piss of farm animals) released into the air nationwide. Never mind the fact that the EPA names factory farming to be the single largest contributor of polluted American waterways. Factory farmers do not have to submit to EPA monitoring programs.[198] If it pleases them, they can volunteer. How civilized.

Outraged by the EPA's lack of enforcement, opponents point out that the factory farming industry made $3.46 million in campaign contributions, benefiting mostly Republican federal candidates. The NPPC even went so far as to present President Bush with its "Friend of the Pork Producer" award in 2004, thanking him for his help in "shaping environmental policies impacting agriculture." [199] Yeah, um, thanks for that.

Trust No One

Whether you love him or hate him, President Clinton's administration tried to "implement a tough, science-based food inspection system," according to Eric Schlosser, bestselling author of *Fast Food Nation*. Sad to say, however, these attempts were squashed when the Republican party gained control of Congress in 1994. Schlosser revealed, "The meatpacking industry's allies in Congress worked hard to thwart modernization of the nation's meat inspection system. A great deal of effort was spent denying the federal government any authority to recall contaminated meat or impose civil fines on firms that knowingly ship contaminated products. . . . . The Clinton administration backed legislation to provide the USDA with the authority to demand meat recalls and impose civil fines on meatpackers. [But] Republicans in Congress failed to enact not only that bill, but also similar legislation [for four consecutive years.] . . . Under current law, the USDA cannot demand a recall [of contaminated meat.]" Can you fucking believe this? If a company decides voluntarily to recall contaminated meat, "it is under no legal obligation to inform the public—or even health officials—that a recall is taking place." [200]

Now, we don't mean to say that everyone working for the government is evil. Surely there are some decent, caring, moral, intelligent, well-intentioned people working for the FDA, EPA,

USDA, and Bush administration. One former staff attorney-turned-environmentalist said the EPA "hasn't initiated one investigation in four years. They're not doing anything."[201] See, she's a "good guy!" She finked on the EPA. Unfortunately, many of the "good guys" seem to be lost in the shuffle of politics and greed within these groups.

So do yourself a favor and trust no one. Read ingredients. Ignore everything else. And, if you're totally incensed by what you've just learned, do something. Contact your representatives, senators, the President and Vice President and demand reform of these crooked, self-serving agencies. Go to www.congress.org to send a quick e-mail to these politicians. While you're at it, write a letter to the editor of your favorite magazine or newspaper, and ask others to join the crusade. Visit www.congress.org and click on "media guide" to access their contact information.

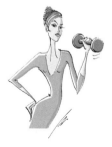

Chapter 10

Don't Be a Pussy

What if someone told you that you could totally change your life and have the body you want for the rest of your life? What if all you had to do was follow a simple formula and maybe struggle for a month or two? What if you could reprogram your brain to actually enjoy healthy foods? Well, guess what? You *can* change your life. You *can* have the body you want for the rest of your life. You *can* enjoy healthy foods. All you have to do is follow a simple formula, and be willing to delay gratification for a few months. A few months. That's it. Then you can enjoy a new body for the *rest of your life.* Don't be a pussy. You have all the nutritional information you need to become a Skinny Bitch. The rest is up to you. While this is a lifestyle, and not a diet, it is going to feel like a diet for the first thirty days or so. During this time, you will be retraining your brain, healing your taste buds, and cleansing and detoxifying your body. It might suck a little. Chances are, there will be times you feel deprived, angry, overwhelmed, and frustrated. But these few, fleeting moments will all be worthwhile once you are skinny. Truth be told, if you follow our guidelines, it won't be so bad.

Before you even start making changes, take notice of how you feel and the role that your diet plays. Do you wake up tired? Is coffee the only thing that gets you going in the morning? Are you cranky in the afternoon? Do you need snacks to bolster your mood? Do you have little or no energy? Do you rely on soda or sugar for a little boost? Do you have trouble falling asleep? Is a glass of wine the only thing that gets you drowsy? When you eat something unhealthy, how do you feel while you're eating it? Right after? An hour later? How does it affect your sleep that night? How do you feel the next day? Pay attention to the negative effects your current diet and lifestyle have on your body, moods, and energy level. Feel free to start a little journal, writing what you eat and drink throughout the day and how you feel as a result. This way, when you start making positive changes to your diet, you'll appreciate *all* of the results—not just the weight loss.

Recognize that anything worth having is worth fighting for. Good health, vitality, more energy, more confidence, better sex, great abs, a tight ass—you either want 'em or you don't. You can continue plodding along in your life feeling like you're not living up to your glorious potential or you can dedicate yourself to creating the life you want. Fuck excuses about not having the time or the money. You spend forty hours a week working, or more if you're a full-time mom. Certainly your health and your body and *you* are more important than anything else in your life. You are worthless to your colleagues, friends, and family if you do not value yourself enough to take excellent care of *you*. Yes, you have to put *yourself* before your friends, parents, boyfriend, husband, and even your children. It won't make you a bad daughter or wife or mother; it will make you a less resentful, more confident, interesting, beautiful, patient, tolerant, and fun person to be around. Your bright, shining light will give everyone around you the permission and inspiration to shine more brightly. Love yourself enough to do whatever it takes to be the best *you* you can be.

An important part of any recovery program for addiction—and unhealthy eating is an addiction—is taking one day at a time. Don't torture yourself with thoughts of, "I can never eat steak again," or "How will I live without coffee?" Just take it one meal at a time. Don't think ahead with dread and anguish. One meal at a time. And when all feels hopeless, remember that you are in charge of what goes into your body, you don't answer to anyone, and you are *allowed* to eat anything you want. Often just knowing we *can* eat whatever we want is enough to keep us from eating whatever we want. We're so rebellious.

If you feel really invigorated and motivated, and you're ready to completely immerse yourself in the Skinny Bitch lifestyle now, then rock on. Go for it. Otherwise, feel free to set mini-goals for yourself and tackle them one at a time. This means, spend the first week of your new life removing one dirty vice item. Whether it's cigarettes or coffee or alcohol or sugar or junk food or meat or dairy—just purge something negative from your life immediately. Choose something that you like and enjoy, but that you know you can let go of successfully. (But start right now. Don't let these intense feelings fade—use them.) Dedicate the week to getting this vice item out of your diet, your body, your kitchen, and your mind. Think of all you've learned about this item, and how disgusting it is. Envision the damaging effect it has on your organs, your mood, your health, and your appearance. Imagine exactly what it is that you'd be eating. Know how shitty you'd feel, physically and mentally, if you ate it. Understand that you have free will and that if you *wanted* to eat it, you could. But know with every fiber and cell of your being that *today* you wish to put only pure, beautiful, healthful foods in your body. Most important, acknowledge that no vice item will ever make you feel happy or whole or satisfied. In fact, all vice items make you *unhappy* because they contribute to weight issues, health problems, mood swings, and low self-esteem.

When you've got one week under your belt, feel great about what you've accomplished. Then, immediately, while continuing to steer clear of the item you banished in week one, start week two by ridding something else from your diet. Every week, until you've completely cleansed your life of poison and toxins, eliminate one more thing. Apply the same mindset, dedication, technique, and excitement you used in week one. Resign yourself to purifying your thoughts, body, and kitchen of this crappy vice item; realize you've just made your life better by not letting this vice item infect you anymore; gross yourself out thinking about what exactly it is and the effects it has on your body; think of how bad it makes you feel when you partake in it; and finally, remember that if you did *choose* to eat/smoke/drink it, it wouldn't make you happy or fulfilled.

Never feel like or say you are "giving up" your favorite foods. Those words have a negative connotation, like you are sacrificing something. You're not *giving up* anything. You are simply empowered now and able to make educated, controlled choices about what you will and won't put into your body, your temple. Be grateful that you now know the truth about the foods you used to poison yourself with. Let all you think and speak of regarding this life change be positive. People who have positive attitudes are much more successful than those who don't. Be excited about feeling clean, pure, healthy, energized, happy, and skinny. Enjoy every second of this metamorphosis, knowing the journey is as important as the end result.

Confucius never said, "A hungry woman is like a tornado of red ants and wildebeasts," but he should have. Because it's true. A hungry woman is a crazy woman, who will destroy everything in her path to be rid of the hunger. So you must always be prepared with healthy food on hand. Otherwise, seriously, you will fall off the wagon almost immediately. Your kitchen should be stocked at all times with the appropriate foods. Pack your lunch and a snack for school or work. Keep an emergency stash in your car, at your desk, and in your purse. Never, ever get caught with your pants down. Unfortunately, depending on where you live, restaurants may not be a safe place for the first month. The menu might not have any vegan or even vegetarian options, and it is easy to be hypnotized by the seductive smells of cooking. This doesn't mean you can't eat out ever again as long as you live. Just for thirty days. (Unless there are good veggie-friendly restaurants in your neighborhood.) You can't expect to change your life without a few minor adjustments. Your only priority for thirty days is to adhere to the regimen you're creating. Without straying. After you achieve thirty days of pure eating, you'll feel confident you have what it takes to get the job done. "I just survived thirty days. I'm so proud of myself. This is the healthiest I've ever been in my whole life. If I *want* to, I can eat an old vice item. But why would I? I just made it thirty consecutive days. I'm going to keep going." If you test yourself before thirty days, you are setting yourself up for failure. Be patient and strong.

When you reach the thirty-day milestone, don't run out and gorge yourself on crap. In fact, just keep doing what you've been doing. See and feel all the positive changes in your body, energy level, and self-esteem. Alcohol, cigarettes, coffee, and food are all addictive, physically and psychologically. Chances are, even after the thirty days, if you indulge in a vice item, you might go off the deep end. It is well known in Alcoholics Anonymous that you're only "one drink away from your next drunk." This means we think we can control our addictions. "I'll just have one drink. I'll just have pizza this one time. I'll just eat half a piece of cake." The truth of the matter is that we are powerless over our addictions. We don't want to make you feel like you can never eat your favorite foods ever again. We just want to impress upon you that it is very easy to obliterate all your progress with one bite, sip, or puff.

Anyway, after one month of pure living, if you did eat the food you've been fantasizing about, you probably wouldn't even enjoy it. Really. You'd see that your brain has been tricking you and your taste buds all along. Now that your taste buds have healed and become more sensitized and your brain knows the truth, those old chemical, sugary, artificial, dead, rotting foods will taste "off" or "less than" somehow.

If you do decide to partake in a vice item after thirty days, it cannot be out of weakness or for lack of preparation. You should never be somewhere and just say, "Fuck it." It should be a calculated, scheduled, premeditated choice. The portion should be decided on beforehand, should be smaller than you would normally have had, and served on a plate. (The package should be put away before you start eating.) Sit down at a table. Eat very slowly. Try not to finish the whole thing. Do not have another serving. Take note of how you feel while you're eating it, immediately after, an hour later, in bed that night, and the next day. Chances are, because your body is now pure, the vice item will make you feel a little nauseous, or headache-y, at the very least. And it most certainly won't taste as good as you imagine it will. Do not discount these negative feelings. They are your new, healthy, clean, pure organs speaking to you.

Enough of all this melodrama. It's not like you're gonna be hungry and cranky for all of eternity. We know that dieters always "crash" when their favorite foods become forbidden. So we devised the Skinny Bitch plan to allow for cookies, cakes, chocolate, burgers, ice cream, etc. They just aren't the same ones you're used to. You're not giving up anything; you're just trading in all your old, gross food. Big deal. The new stuff is just as good. So don't kid yourself with the old "I had a craving" routine. Nobody's buying it.

The only thing more annoying than the "Where do you get your protein?" question is the "My body is craving meat, I must need iron" comment. Most cravings are not reliable indicators of what your body needs. Smokers crave cigarettes, alcoholics crave alcohol, drug addicts crave drugs, and junk food eaters crave junk. If you eat shit for a few days, and you begin to crave a salad or a piece of fruit, that's a craving you can trust. Otherwise, it's just your addiction talking. Bitch-slap it, and get a hold of yourself. But feel free to try and understand your addiction first.

In order for us to survive, our brains came equipped with dopamine, a pleasure-producing chemical. Dopamine is released during sex (or even just while flirting), so that we procreate and the human race won't die out. And food stimulates dopamine release so that we'll remember to eat and nourish our bodies. Basically, anything the brain perceives to be enjoyable will cause dopamine to lock onto brain cells and build a permanent memory trace of where pleasure comes from. Even though this evolved out of the need for survival, sometimes this can be a bad thing. Heroin, cocaine, alcohol, and nicotine all trigger the brain's pleasure circuitry. And not surprisingly, chocolate, sugar, and cheese also affect this same part of the brain. So you see, we can be *physiologically* addicted to food. Any food can trigger the brain's pleasure center. Some of us are fortunate enough to experience dopamine ecstasy while eating broccoli, and we actually crave this healthy food. But the types of food and the degree of pleasure they bring will differ from one person to the next. The trick is resetting our memory traces to feel pleasure from healthy food, and no pleasure from junk food.[202]

Easier said than done. Especially for people who are addicted to cigarettes, alcohol, or drugs, or are overweight. Studies have shown that these people have fewer receptors for dopamine than other people. For them, the pleasure-giving chemical has fewer places to attach to brain cells, making it difficult for them to experience pleasurable feelings. So, because they aren't getting that "pleasure rush," they tend to smoke, drink, use drugs, gamble, or overeat. Now don't automatically diagnose yourself as one these people and assume you'll never get healthy. We are not at the mercy of our bodies. We are the commanders of our bodies.[203]

Unless we eat cheese. Cheese will rule our lives and fatten our asses if we don't kick the addiction. Cow's milk actually has traces of morphine in it! And for once, we can't blame factory farming. Morphine, along with codeine and other opiates, are naturally produced in cows' livers and end up in their milk. But that's not all. All milk, whether from a cow or a human, contains *casein,* a protein that breaks apart during digestion and releases a whole slew of opiates. All these "feel good" chemicals exist so that newborns will nurse and thrive, and to ensure a bond between mothers and their young.[204]

Are you starting to get the picture? When a woman breastfeeds, her milk has an almost drug-like effect on the baby. The baby is totally hooked. He'll cry, not because he's hungry, but because he needs "a fix" of that pleasurable feeling produced by the opiates. Nature has guaranteed that our babies will nurse and grow. And when they reach a certain age, we wean them, and stop giving them these "drugs." And they're fine. But then we start them on cows' milk and an addiction is born.

All dairy products contain casein, but cheese has the highest concentration. In fact, cheese contains far more casein than is naturally found in cows' milk. It also has phenylethylamine (PEA), an amphetamine-like chemical. So when we kid around and say, "I am addicted to cheese," it's not a joke—it's true. We are chemically addicted to cheese.[205]

Casein even finds its way into soy cheese. Whether manufacturers use it to up the protein content, to aide in melting, or because they know of its addictive quality, casein still has the same effect. So if you see casein on the list of ingredients, run! (Follow Your Heart's Vegan Gourmet cheeses are casein-free and totally vegan, so enjoy.)

The following hormones and natural chemicals have all been identified in cows' milk: prolactin, somatostatin, melatonin, oxytocin, growth hormone, leuteinizing hormone-releasing hormone, thyrotropin-releasing hormone, thyroid-stimulating hormone, vasoactive intestinal peptide, calcitonin, parathyroid hormone, corticosteroids, estrogens, progesterone, insulin, epidermal growth

factor, insulin-like growth factor, erythropoietin, bombesin, neu-
rotensin, motilin, and cholecystokinin.[206] If you think your will is
strong enough to conquer all those mother-fuckers, you're on
drugs! Dairy is fattening,[207] and if you eat it, you'll never get skinny.
You cannot control your addiction. You can't "just have one slice of
pizza," or "only have cheese at parties." You're only one piece-of-
cheese away from a total relapse. Eat the substitutes; they'll get you
through.

Thankfully, our bodies produce a few different chemical substances that help tame our appetites. One such hormone, leptin, is
made by our fat cells. When fat cells in our bodies get adequate
nourishment, they release leptin into the blood for two purposes.
The first task at hand is alerting the brain to diminish the appetite.
Next, our metabolism gets boosted, encouraging the body's cells to
burn calories more quickly. Pretty cool, huh? Until we start "diet-
ing." Typical low-calorie diets confuse the body into thinking it's
starving. So our fat cells slow down their leptin production, to help
increase our appetites. Release the hounds! Now, we feel like we're
starving! So we trash our diets and binge like rabid beasts. But diets
high in fat don't fare any better. Fatty diets (think animal products)

also lower leptin levels. You know where this is headed: Low-fat, plant-based diets actually boost leptin levels, helping each molecule of leptin to work more effectively. So help yourself succeed. Eating healthy foods like fruits, vegetables, whole grains, and beans will help curb your appetite and stimulate your metabolism.[208]

But when we have PMS, all bets are off. There's no telling when we'll cry, whom we'll kill, or what we'll eat. One culprit of mood swings and cravings is estrogen. Every month, our bodies produce extra estrogen in case of pregnancy. When we don't become preggers, estrogen levels plunge, triggering bloating, irritability, and cravings. The trick to avoiding these heinous feelings is maintaining balanced estrogen levels throughout the month. Like everything else, this can be done through diet. Fatty foods increase estrogen levels, while fibrous foods help reduce estrogen production. The *Journal of Obstetrics and Gynecology* conducted a study exploring the effects of diet on menstrual symptoms. Women who eliminated animal fats from their diets experienced dramatic decreases of bloating and cravings. On average, menstrual cramps were reduced from four days to about two and a half days.[209] Less cramps, cravings, and bloating! Those reasons alone are enough to swear off animal products.

Even if you do have some serious PMS cravings, the good thing about the Skinny Bitch regimen is that there are plenty of naughty-tasting foods that you don't need to feel bad about. So eat all day long. As long as everything you put in your mouth meets Skinny Bitch approval, it's fine. Just be sure that when you're full, you *stop eating*. We know this is a foreign concept, but we're hoping it'll catch on. Imagine the actual size of your stomach (about the size of a one-quart container) or imagine what size you want it to be. There is no need to cram it full and stretch the shit out of it three times a day, every day, for your entire life. Look at the portion you put on your plate. Do you think it will fit in your stomach nicely, or that you'll need to force it in? Pare down.

Just because you're "starving," you don't need to eat faster. When you're done eating, if you have the hiccups, indigestion, a stomachache, or you're burping and farting, that means you're eating too fast and gulping down air. Slow down. Breathe evenly. Conversely, make sure you aren't holding your breath while you speed-eat. It takes time for your brain to get the message that your stomach is full. The slower you eat, the less likely you are to overeat. Also, be sure to chew your food purposefully and slowly. Rest in between bites. Do not watch TV, read a magazine, talk on the phone, or do *anything else* while you are eating. The goal is to know when you're full (without having *stuffed* yourself) and be able to put the fork down. You aren't six anymore. You won't get the praise of elders for cleaning your plate. It's okay to leave food on your plate.

But if you do still get off on scoring brownie points, you can earn extra credit by fasting. Yeah, fasting—willfully abstaining from food. For more than five thousand years, fasting has been used as a healthy method of weight loss. It is also a powerful tool for cleaning, flushing, detoxifying, and maintaining the body, and healing illnesses, both minor and major.[210] When we eat, all of our body's energy goes toward digesting, using, and storing the food, and eliminating the waste. When we don't eat, all of our body's energy goes toward cleaning house. And with all the years of abuse, our house could sure use a cleaning. We absorb toxic chemicals from food, drinks, and the environment. Our body eliminates some of these through waste, but the rest remain as chemical by-products and free radicals (highly reactive chemicals that damage cells and contribute to premature aging, heart disease, and cancer). Fasting gets rid of these toxins. It also increases our blood's white cell count, which boosts immunity and protects us from disease. And because fasting is beneficial for the circulatory system, you can expect better skin, hair, and nails.[211]

Fasts can last anywhere from twenty-four hours to ten days or more. It's all up to you and how light, clean, and healthy you want to get. The longer the better, but even just one day one time a month is beneficial. There are too many types of fasts to cover them all, so we'll explain just a few. But it is imperative to really read up on fasting before diving in.

A particular favorite is a raw or "live" food fast, when, obviously, you eat only raw foods for however many days you choose. This is a great beginner's fast, because you reap the benefits of fasting, while still being able to actually eat. It's also a good fast to do if you want to work your way up to a more stringent fast, like a juice fast, where the only thing you put in your body is fresh-pressed or fresh-squeezed juice (not pasteurized or packaged). Whether its fruit juice, veggie juice, or both, the enzymes are wonderful aides in the cleansing process. A liquid fast is similar to the juice fast, but includes soups,

too (no beans or rice or chunks—just liquid). The alkalizing properties of the juices and soups help to neutralize the toxins being
released from the body.[212] For this and other reasons, the hardest fast
is a water fast, where you have nothing but water. Don't be a competitive ass and launch yourself into this fast from the diet you exist on
now. You've gotta learn to crawl before you can walk.

Most people like to ease into a fast. They might eat smaller portions for a week prior. Or if they usually eat vegan junk food, they
might abstain in preparation. We highly recommend eating as pure-
ly as possible leading up to a fast. (Meat-eaters should go
vegetarian and then vegan before fasting.) It makes the transition
more gradual and less jarring. Regardless of which fast you choose,
be sure to drink a lot of water throughout. Your body will be detox-
ing like crazy, and you don't want to become dehydrated.

All fasts are challenging, both physically and mentally. Do not
expect it to be easy, especially at the beginning when you find yourself salivating over foods you don't normally even care about. But
eventually, you get to a place where you are truly not hungry, and
you feel light, clean, pure, and divine. When you do reintroduce
food back into your diet, which should be done slowly with great

care, you are almost repulsed by things you previously ate. It is quite beautiful to have such a new, fresh perspective. It is a real gift to see truths that weren't apparent before. Periodic repeated fasts are especially useful for this reason. They help our bodies and minds reestablish a new relationship with food. In fact, because of this, fasting can even be used to overcome addictions. When we eliminate the toxins that cause "cell memory cravings," we can eradicate the need for the food or drug that provided those toxins.[213]

Not surprisingly, some people experience headaches, weakness, nausea, cramping, stomach pains, sweating, a swollen tongue, bad breath, general aches and pains, increased temperature, or depression while fasting.[214] Abstaining from food does not *cause* these ailments. They are simply normal side effects of fasting. After two to three days of fasting, the body goes into autolysis, and actually starts digesting its own cells. With its wisdom, the body selectively decomposes the tissues and cells that are diseased, damaged, old, dead or in excess (fat).[215] The body is literally digesting and expelling poisons, toxins, and bad cells that were already there—and it feels crappy. But this is actually a good thing, because the body is finally able to tackle some problems that were lurking within.

During a fast, digestive enzymes are relieved from their usual role, and instead act to cleanse and rejuvenate the body. This rejuvenation process includes the production of new cells. And when more cells are being produced than are dying, the aging process is actually being reversed. This phenomenon occurs during juice and water fasts. Eventually, you'll notice sharper senses of smell, sight, sound, and taste. You'll feel lighter physically, mentally, and emotionally.[216]

All magic aside, fasting is *not* for you if you're pregnant, lactating, underweight, or suffering from severe wasting diseases, such as neurological degenerative diseases and certain cancers. Diabetics and people suffering from hypoglycemia can fast, but only with medical supervision.[217] For that matter, anyone with any medical condition should consult a doctor before fasting.

Vitamins

Vitamins are an integral part of a healthy lifestyle. Here are some significant vitamins and minerals, a description of why they're important, and which foods provide them:

Calcium strengthens bones, provides for healthy teeth, reduces risk of colon cancer, decreases chances of bone loss, aids the nervous system, and alleviates insomnia. Eat almonds, Brazil nuts, seeds, nuts, soybeans, kale, collard greens, broccoli, kelp, and molasses to get calcium.

Folic acid promotes healthy skin, protects against parasites and food poisoning, helps ward off anemia, and fights against birth defects. To get folic acid, eat leafy green veggies, carrots, artichokes, fruit, cantaloupe, avocados, apricots, beans, lentils, soybeans, garbanzos, barley, and whole wheat.

Iron aids growth, promotes resistance to disease, prevents fatigue and anemia, and enhances good skin tone. It can be found in nuts, pumpkin seeds, beans, lentils, whole grains, oatmeal, asparagus, molasses, broccoli, spinach, bok choy, peas, swiss chard, green beans, and sea veggies.

Magnesium (known as the anti-stress mineral) fights depression, boosts energy, helps burn fat, prevents heart attacks, maintains good cholesterol levels, aids indigestion, combats PMS symptoms, helps prevent premature labor, and keeps teeth strong and healthy. When combined with calcium, it works as a natural tranquilizer. Eat nuts, seeds, sunflower seeds, green

vegetables, soybeans, kelp (seaweed), and molasses to get a
good dose, especially if you're on The Pill.

Omega-3 fatty acids fight heart disease, lower bad cholesterol
levels, lessen the likelihood of blood clots, reduce the risk of
breast cancer, help with rheumatoid arthritis, and keep skin,
hair, and nails healthy. Sources for these fatty acids are
flaxseeds, walnuts, pumpkin seeds, hempseed oil, and other
seeds and their unrefined oils.

Omega-6 fatty acids combat PMS, ward off acne, eczema, and pso-
riasis, and help with endometriosis and rheumatoid arthritis.
Flaxseed oil, evening primrose oil, borage oil, and black cur-
rant seed oil are all good sources.

Potassium aids in reducing blood pressure, increases clear thinking by helping send oxygen to the brain, and helps the body
dispose of waste. It's found in bananas, citrus fruits, cantaloupe, tomatoes, watercress, green leafy vegetables,
sunflower seeds, avocados, lentils, potatoes, and whole
grains.

The **B Vitamins** improve mental attitude, aid in digestion, help
migraine headaches, contribute to healthy skin, act as natural

diuretics, strengthen immunity, increase energy, improve concentration and memory, and are good for the nervous system.
Eat whole wheat, wheat germ, bran, oatmeal, whole grains,
brown rice, beans, nuts, seeds, soybeans, lentils, dates, figs,
bananas, and vegetables.

Vitamin C accelerates healing, lowers blood pressure, prevents
colds, protects against cancer, and helps decrease blood cholesterol. It also forms collagen, which is important for growth
the and repair tissue cells, blood vessels, gums, bones, and
teeth. Vitamin C is especially important for women who
smoke or take birth control pills. It's easy to get vitamin C by
eating broccoli, brussel sprouts, cabbage, collard greens,
green peppers, spinach, watercress, potatoes, grapefruits,
oranges, and papayas.

Vitamin D, in conjunction with calcium and phosphorous, helps
build strong bones and teeth. Not only does vitamin D help
our bodies assimilate vitamin A, but it also prevents colds
when teamed up with vitamins A and C. All you need to do to
obtain vitamin D is get direct sun exposure on your skin.

Vitamin E keeps you looking younger, inhibits cancer cell growth, fights fatigue, prevents blood clots, lowers blood pressure, decreases the risk of Alzheimer's disease, and accelerates the healing of burns. It's found in wheat germ, whole grain cereals, whole wheat, nuts, sunflower seeds, leafy greens, and vegetable oils.

Zinc helps with infertility issues, is important for brain function, maintains the body's acid/alkaline balance, aids in collagen formation, and helps form insulin (needed for many vital enzymes). Foods with high concentrations of zinc are wheat germ, whole grains, pumpkin seeds, sesame seeds, and soybeans.[218]

When we eat properly, we can get almost all of the nutrients we need from food sources. However, Vitamin B-12 is only found in animal products, so most vegans and vegetarians take B-12 supplements. Sublingual liquid B vitamins with folic acid are more easily and quickly absorbed than pills. If you are concerned that you aren't getting sufficient vitamins in your diet and wish to take supplements, consult a holistic physician.

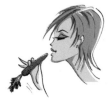

Chapter 11

Let's Eat

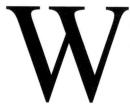e set out to write this book for a few reasons:
- We could not tolerate the cruelty associated with a meat-eating diet and we wanted to help end animal suffering.
- We couldn't bear to have "real" jobs.
- We wanted to change peoples' lives.

We *truly* want to help you succeed and make this all as easy as possible.

In this chapter, we've compiled a few lists so that there will be no confusion as to what you should or shouldn't eat. After reading the whole book, if you're feeling uncertain about what to buy or order, just whip out your little *Skinny Bitch* and come right to this chapter. There will be no doubt that you're making the right food choices.

Breakfast is the most important meal of the day. But not why you think. The cereal and dairy industries lead us to believe that without a big, "healthy" breakfast, we won't have enough energy to get us through the day. But Sugar Smacks with cow's milk hardly constitutes a healthy, viable energy source. The *real* reason breakfast is so important is that it sets the tone for your entire day of eating. If you eat a shitty breakfast, you will likely crave (and eat) crap all day. And, if you eat too early in the morning, you'll be interrupting your body's cleaning session. Remember, when your body isn't working on food, it's working on you! When your "cleaning crew" is in the middle of cleanup, and you start cramming food in, "they" get overwhelmed. They stop what they're doing, throw their hands up, scratch their heads, and finally, decide that they just can't deal with this mess you're making. So they opt to store it away as fat and pretend they'll get to it later.[219] So when you wake up, you should wait to eat breakfast until you're truly hungry. Don't just eat right away because that's what you're used to. After a few days, you'll grow to love that empty feeling in your stomach and know that the initial headaches, nausea, and hunger were just your body's cleaning crew. Feel free to enjoy a cup of caffeine-free, organic, herbal tea upon waking. But other than that, the best thing to do is wait until you're really hungry.

When you do eat, the breakfast of skinny bitches is organic fruit. This may seem light in comparison to your previous bagel or eggs or cereal. But again, once you adapt, you will be totally fulfilled by fruit. Eat one piece (or serving) slowly. After a period of time—perhaps ten minutes or so—when you feel hungry, eat another piece, slowly. When you feel hungry again, eat one more. Breakfast is over.

Breakfast Food List

We hope you'll at least try having just fruit for breakfast before deciding it's not for you. But if you give it a go, and after two weeks you still feel angry and violent just thinking about it, consult our list of acceptable breakfast foods:(R) found in refrigerator section, (F) found in freezer section

Arrowhead Mills: organic blue corn pancake and waffle mix

Arrowhead Mills: organic whole grain pancake and waffle mix

Food For Life: Ezekiel 4:9 cereal

Barbara's Bakery: Puffins cereal

Barbara's Bakery: Shredded Spoonfuls cereal

Peace Cereal: vanilla almond crisp

Peace Cereal: maple pecan crisp

Nature's Path: Optimum Slim cereal

Nature's Path: Optimum Power Breakfast cereal

Health Valley: organic raisin bran flakes

Health Valley: organic oat bran flakes with raisins

Old Wessex Ltd.: Irish-style oatmeal

Old Wessex Ltd.: 5-grain cereal

Nature's Path: organic instant hot maple nut oatmeal

Ancient Harvest: organic quinoa flakes

Rice Dream: original enriched rice milk

Original EdenSoy: organic soymilk

Original EdenBlend: rice & soy beverage

House: tofu steak (R)

Whole Soy & Co.: creamy cultured soy (yogurt) (R)

Silk: cultured soy (yogurt) (R)

Amy's: organic tofu scramble (F)

Van's: all natural organic original waffles (F)

Lifestream: Mesa Sunrise toaster waffles (F)

French Meadow Bakery: men's bread

French Meadow Bakery: healthy hemp sprouted bread

French Meadow Bakery: brown rice bread

Nature's Path: organic Manna breads (F)

Fabe's All Natural Bakery: vegan muffins (F)

Zen Bakery: muffins (R)

Zen Bakery: cinnamon raisin rolls (R)

Whole Foods: organic English muffins (R)

Food For Life: Ezekiel 4:9 sprouted grain bagels (F)

Tofutti: Better Than Cream Cheese (R) (the kind *without* hydrogenated oils.)

Lightlife: Smart Bacon (R)

Lightlife: Gimme Lean! sausage style (R)

Organic Fruit: (Earlier, we mentioned the benefit of eating just fruit for breakfast. But here, we did include other breakfast foods.

It is up to you to decide how diligent you want to be with your diet. We just wanted to provide hearty breakfast choices should you disregard the fruit-by-itself theory. Totally your choice. You can eat the fruit before eating the muffin or pancakes or waffles. Whatever you want.)

Lunch Food List

Don't eat lunch until you're close to ravenous. This will allow your breakfast to pass through your body without having food piled on top of it. In a perfect, skinny world, lunch consists of a fresh, organic salad with lots of raw vegetables. But if that's too boring or stringent for you, feel free to choose something else from our yummy lunch list:

Food For Life: Ezekiel 4:9 bread (F) (or bakery/bread aisle)

Arrowhead Mills: organic Valencia peanut butter

MaraNatha: organic raw almond butter

I.M. Healthy: SoyNut butter

Bionaturae: organic fruit spreads

Natural Touch: Tuno (faux tuna)

Morningstar Farms: Tuno

Amy's: All American burger (F)

Amy's: California burger (F)

Amy's: Texas burger (F)

Gardenburger's: flame-grilled burgers (F)

Gardenburger's: flame-grilled chik'n (F)

Whole Foods Bakehouse: organic burger buns

Tofurkey: deli slices

Yves: veggie bologna (R)

Yves: veggie turkey (R)

Yves: veggie salami (R)

Follow Your Heart: Vegan Gourmet cheese alternative (R)

Earthbound Farm: organic salad greens (R)

Fantastic Foods: tabouli

Fantastic Foods: organic whole wheat couscous

Fantastic Carb 'Tastic Soup: vegetarian chicken gumbo

Fantastic Carb 'Tastic Soup: shiitake mushroom

Fantastic Big Soup: five bean

Fantastic Big Soup: country lentil

Amy's Organic Soups: black bean vegetable

Amy's Organic Soups: butternut squash

Amy's Organic Soups: lentil vegetable

Amy's Organic Soups: chunky vegetable

Amy's: organic chili

Health Valley: organic split pea soup

Health Valley: organic lentil soup

Health Valley: organic black bean soup

Imagine: organic vegetable broth

Imagine: organic no-chicken broth

Pacific: organic vegetable broth

organic vegetables

Dinner Food List

When you're feeling really hungry, it's time for din-din. Dinner is easy and fun. Just pick from the list, or create your own healthy vegan fest:

Health Best 100% Organic: red lentils

Health Best 100% Organic: green lentils

Health Best 100% Organic: barley

Health Best 100% Organic: split peas

Health Best 100% Organic: amaranth

Arrowhead Mills: organic whole millet

Lundberg Family Farms: organic short grain brown rice

Lundberg Family Farms: organic brown rice pasta

DeBoles: organic whole wheat pasta

Ancient Harvest: organic quinoa supergrain pasta

Eddie's Spaghetti: organic vegetable pasta

Pastariso: organic brown rice fettuccine

Pastariso: organic brown rice elbow macaroni

Rising Moon Organics: spinach Florentine ravioli with tofu (F)

Chef Nikola's Kitchen: roasted eggplant in herbed balsamic sauce
     (F)

Amy's Organic: Asian noodle stir-fry (F)

Amy's Organic: Thai stir-fry (F)

Amy's: roasted vegetable pizza (no cheese) (F)

Nate's: meatless meatballs (F)

Health is Wealth: buffalo wings (F)

Health is Wealth: chicken-free patties (F)

Health is Wealth: chicken-free nuggets (F)

Tofurkey: *Tofurkey* dinner (F)

Gloria's Kitchen: assorted vegan prepared entrees (F)

Lightlife: organic tempeh (R)

Lightlife: *Smart Ground* (ground "meat") (F)

Nasoya: organic tofu (R)

White Wave: chicken-style seitan (R)

Lightlife: *Smart Dogs* (R)

Yves: veggie dogs (R)

Rudi's Organic Bakery: white hot dog rolls

Now & Zen: *UnChicken* (R)

Now & Zen: *UnSteak* (R)

Yves: *Veggie Ground Round Mexican* (Mexican-style ground "meat") (F)

Bearitos: taco shells

Garden of Eatin': blue corn taco shells

Alvarado St. Bakery: organic sprouted wheat tortillas

organic vegetables

Obviously, the foods on the lunch and dinner lists can be used interchangeably.

A helpful hint: Prepare large batches of staple food items on

Sunday night, to tide you over for your busy workweek. Brown rice, lentils, homemade hummus, soups, and pastas are all good candidates. But try not to do this with your veggies because they'll lose some of their enzymatic punch.

Acceptable Junk Food, Snacks & Desserts

There's something about a snack that makes you feel like a kid again. And that's a good thing. If you're hungry, but not quite ready for dinner, have a small snack. As long as it's healthy, it doesn't spoil your dinner, and you only have a small serving, there is no reason to feel bad about having a snickety-snack. But don't have one just because you can. Only eat it if you want it. Otherwise, just wait for dinner.

Dessert is one of God's many gifts to humans. Indulge. Like snacks, if your desserts are healthy and eaten in controlled portions, enjoy them without the guilt!

365: organic chocolate soymilk

Whole Foods: organic date coconut rolls

Barbara's Bakery: organic graham crackers

Dagoba: organic dark chocolate bars

Uncle Eddie's: vegan cookies

Organica Foods: vegan cookies

Fabe's All Natural Bakery: vegan cookies

Newman's Own: organic Fig Newmans

Laura's Wholesome Junk Food: *Bitelettes* (cookies)

Nutrilicious Natural Bakery: donut holes

MI-DEL: vanilla snaps

Country Choice: certified organic sandwich cremes

Back to Nature: classic creme sandwich cookies

Back to Nature: chocolate & mint creme sandwich cookies

Chocolove: Belgian dark chocolate

Endangered Species: dark chocolate bars

Tropical Source: rice crisp dark chocolate

Ecco Bella: *Health By Chocolate*

Raw Balance: *Carobelles* (www.rawbalance.com)

Gertrude & Bronner's Magic: *Alpsnack*

LäraBar: all flavors

Terra: exotic vegetable chips original

Terra: spiced sweet potato chips

Maine Coast Sea Vegetables: sea chips

Garden of Eatin': *Sunny Blues* (tortilla chips with sunflower seeds)

Guiltless Gourmet: yellow corn baked chips

Kettle Organic Tortilla Chips: sesame blue moons

Veggie Stix: shoestring potato sticks

Robert's American Gourmet: *Tings*

Robert's American Gourmet: *Spicy Tings*

Robert's American Gourmet: *Veggie Booty*

Newman's Own: organic salted round pretzels

Koyo Organic Rice Cakes: dulse

Koyo Organic Rice Cakes: mixed grain

Nature's Path: tamari flax crackers

Back to Nature: classic rounds

Soy Dream: non-dairy frozen desserts (F)

Soy Delicious: non-dairy frozen desserts (F)

Double Rainbow Soy Cream: non-dairy desserts (F)

Soy Delicious: *Li'l Buddies* ("ice cream" sandwiches) (F)

Sweet Nothings: non-dairy fudge bars (F)

Condiments, Baking Supplies & Miscellaneous

Don't worry about the little odds and ends. We've thought of everything.

Earth Balance: natural buttery spread (R)

Soy Garden: natural buttery spread (R)

Follow Your Heart: *Vegenaise* (mayonnaise substitute) (R)

Nasoya: *Nayonaise*

Muir Glen: organic ketchup

Westbrae: natural ketchup

Whole Kids: organic yellow mustard

Spectrum Naturals: organic sesame oil

Spectrum Naturals: organic canola oil

Spectrum Naturals: organic extra virgin olive oil

MaraNatha: organic raw tahini

Bragg Liquid Aminos: all purpose seasoning (soy sauce substitute)

Sea Seasonings: organic kelp granules with cayenne

Annie's Naturals: goddess dressing

OrganicVille: sesame tamari organic vinaigrette

The Wizard's: organic original vegetarian Worcestershire sauce

Essential Living Foods: organic agave nectar or syrup

Shady Maple Farms: certified organic pure maple syrup

Sugar in the Raw: Turbinado sugar from natural cane

Florida Crystals: organic cane sugar

Wholesome Sweeteners: organic sucanat

Hain Pure Foods: organic brown sugar

Stevita Company Inc.: stevia spoonable

Dr. Oetker Organics: chocolate cake mix

Dr. Oetker Organics: vanilla cake mix

Dr. Oetker Organics: chocolate icing mix

Dr. Oetker Organics: vanilla icing mix

Dr. Oetker Organics: chocolate chip cookie mix

Ener-G: egg replacer

Chatfield's Carob & Compliments: dairy-free carob morsels

Sunspire: grain-sweetened chocolate chips

Arrowhead Mills: organic oat flour

Arrowhead Mills: organic whole wheat flour

Arrowhead Mills: organic spelt flour

Arrowhead Mills: organic brown rice flour

Arrowhead Mills: organic blue corn meal
Arrowhead Mills: organic yellow corn meal
Arrowhead Mills: organic flax seeds

When crafting your own day of eating from the food lists provided, use your head. Create a well-balanced menu for the day without being repetitive. For example, don't eat pancakes for breakfast, a sandwich for lunch, and a soy burger for dinner. That would be eating all bread, but no fruits or veggies. Duh. Use your head. Try to always think in terms of fruits, veggies, whole grains, soy, and legumes for a well-balanced day of eating.

If you need a little more guidance, feast your eyes on this, a month's worth of menus:

Week One

Monday

Breakfast: Mango, banana, kiwi and soy yogurt.
Lunch: Spinach salad with shredded carrots, chopped almonds, red onion, fresh garlic, cubed tofu, and sesame oil.

Dinner: Pasta with zucchini, tomatoes, garlic, fresh parsley, pine nuts, and olive oil.

Tuesday

Breakfast: Fresh squeezed orange juice, whole grain muffin with soy butter, banana, and strawberries.

Lunch: Tabouli salad with marinated tofu, eggplant, and red peppers.

Dinner: Veggie nachos! Corn chips with veggie chili, soy cheese, guacamole, scallions, and tomatoes.

Wednesday

Breakfast: Fresh squeezed grapefruit juice and slow-cooking oatmeal with blueberries, strawberries, and raspberries.

Lunch: Veggie burger on whole grain bun with red onion, lettuce, tomato, avocado, and alfalfa sprouts. Served with vegan potato salad.

Dinner: Fake chicken patty with brown rice, lentils, and steamed kale.

Thursday

Breakfast: Fresh squeezed OJ, whole grain bagel with vegan cream cheese, sliced tomatoes, and red onion.

Lunch: Soup and salad.

Dinner: Veggie stir-fry with peppers, onions, garlic, carrots, bok choy, and mushrooms served with brown rice and tofu.

Friday

Breakfast: Granola with sliced banana, peaches, and blueberries with soy yogurt.

Lunch: Club sandwich with fake bacon, fake turkey slices, avocado, lettuce, tomato, sprouts, and Vegenaise (fake mayo). Served with three-bean salad.

Dinner: Take out from your favorite Thai restaurant: vegan Pad Thai, emphasizing no egg or shrimp or fish stock.

Saturday

Breakfast: Fresh squeezed OJ, blue corn and blueberry pancakes served with fresh strawberries.

Lunch: Salad with shredded carrots, couscous, cranberries, and walnuts, dressed with citrus vinaigrette. Served with lentil soup.

Dinner: Veggie fajitas with sautéed peppers, onions, mushrooms, and fake chicken strips, topped with fresh Pico de Gallo.

Sunday

Breakfast: Fresh squeezed OJ and tofu scramble with zucchini, peppers, onions, garlic, spinach, and kale served with whole grain toast.

Lunch: Lentil salad with asparagus tips and walnuts in a raspberry vinaigrette. Served with an entire steamed artichoke and a vegan lemon-butter dipping sauce.

Dinner: No-cheese or vegan-cheese pizza loaded with veggies!

Week Two

Monday

Breakfast: Fruit smoothie with a splash of OJ and fresh banana, frozen pineapple, and coconut.

Lunch: All-American salad with romaine lettuce, corn, peas, and BBQ tofu cubes in a vegan ranch dressing.

Dinner: Italian night! Your favorite pasta and tomato sauce with fake meatballs and whole grain garlic bread.

Tuesday

Breakfast: Fresh squeezed OJ, cereal with soy or rice milk, served with blueberries, sliced banana, and strawberries.

Lunch: Veggie chili with corn bread!

Dinner: Mashed potatoes, Gardenburger Meatless Riblets, and
sautéed collard greens and Swiss chard.

Wednesday

Breakfast: Fresh squeezed OJ and toaster waffles with sliced strawberries, bananas, and peaches.

Lunch: Vegan Caesar salad with fake chicken chunks.

Dinner: Brown rice and lentils with steamed broccoli and red cabbage.

Thursday

Breakfast: A shitload of cantaloupe.

Lunch: Fake deli meats on whole grain bread with lettuce and tomato
and a side of Asian cole slaw (shredded carrots, red cabbage,
green cabbage, rice vinegar, sesame oil, and sesame seeds).

Dinner: Fake meatloaf served with corn on the cob, peas, and
sautéed spinach and garlic.

Friday

Breakfast: Smoothie time with a splash of apple juice and peaches,
blueberries, raspberries, and a dash of flaxseed oil (or a

tablespoon of ground flaxseeds).

Lunch: Japanese lunch of avocado rolls, miso soup, and a small salad.

Dinner: Veggie burger with sautéed mushrooms, onions, soy cheese, lettuce, and tomato served with baked French "fries."

Saturday

Breakfast: Fresh squeezed OJ and vegan French toast with blueberries, strawberries, and banana.

Lunch: Mixed greens with hearts of palm, sun-dried tomatoes, yellow tomatoes, asparagus, basil, garlic, and pine nuts in an oil and vinegar dressing.

Dinner: Veggie dog loaded with veggie chili and soy cheese, served with vegan potato salad.

Sunday

Breakfast: Fresh squeezed OJ and a fake egg sandwich (using House Tofu Steak extra-firm tofu, sliced and pan fried, with fake bacon and soy cheese on a whole grain bagel with soy butter, salt, pepper, and ketchup).

Lunch: Split pea soup and a mixed greens salad.

Dinner: Penne with butternut squash and raw pesto (pine nuts, basil, garlic, olive oil).

Week Three

Monday

Breakfast: Fresh squeezed OJ and slow-cooking oatmeal with apples, cinnamon, and pecans.

Lunch: Whole-wheat vegetable wrap with sautéed eggplant, portabella mushroom, and roasted red peppers served with a small side salad.

Dinner: Veggie stir-fry with green peppers, carrots, zucchini, tofu, bok choy, onions, and garlic served with brown rice.

Tuesday

Breakfast: A big-ass hunk of honeydew melon.

Lunch: Salad greens with red onion, cherry tomatoes, black beans, and corn, served with a baked sweet potato.

Dinner: Baked Teriyaki tofu with brown jasmine rice and steamed green beans.

Wednesday

Breakfast: Fresh- pressed apple juice and a whole grain bagel with peanut butter, jelly (organic and sugar-free, of course), and sliced banana.

Lunch: Mediterranean platter with hummus, eggplant, grape leaves, falafel, peppers, olives, and tomatoes.

Dinner: Veggie burrito with pinto beans, brown rice, guacamole, soy cheese, lettuce, tomato, and salsa.

Thursday

Breakfast: Granola with bananas, blueberries, strawberries, and soy or rice milk.

Lunch: Portabella mushroom burger with arugula and caramelized onions, served with an avocado-tomato salad.

Dinner: Veggie lasagna with red sauce, your favorite veggies, fake ground meat, and tofu ricotta (in food processor, blend firm tofu, garlic, salt, small amount of olive oil, and dried oregano).

Friday

Breakfast: Fruit salad—go crazy!

Lunch: Fake tuna (Tuno with accents of shredded carrots, chopped onion, diced celery, and Vegenaise) on whole grain bread served with a handful of baked corn chips.

Dinner: Steamed broccoli, carrots, kale, red cabbage, cauliflower, and tofu with brown rice, drizzled with sesame oil and sea salt.

Saturday

Breakfast: Ranchos-fake-Huevos wrap with scrambled tofu, sautéed onions and peppers, black beans, avocado, and salsa in a corn tortilla.

Lunch: Chinese fake chicken salad with snow peas, cabbage, carrots, mandarin oranges, fake chicken chunks, and cashews.

Dinner: Seitan (wheat-meat) with steamed leeks, white beans, and garlic-roasted potatoes.

Sunday

Breakfast: Fresh squeezed OJ and apple cinnamon pancakes with raspberries and bananas.

Lunch: Fake bacon, lettuce, tomato, and avocado on whole grain bread with leftover roasted potatoes from last night's dinner.

Dinner: Veggie shish kabobs with green peppers, red peppers, mushrooms, onions, cherry tomatoes, and Gardenburger Meatless Riblets, served with corn on the cob.

Week Four

Monday

Breakfast: Fruit smoothie with peaches, banana, and strawberries and a splash of soy or rice milk.

Lunch: Chef's salad with mixed greens, carrots, tomatoes, vegan cheese, and assorted chopped fake deli meats.

Dinner: Fake steak with a baked sweet potato, lentils, and steamed kale.

Tuesday

Breakfast: Fresh-squeezed OJ and toaster waffles with banana, strawberries, and blueberries.

Lunch: Veggie minestrone soup with a small side salad.

Dinner: Veggie dog smothered in veggie chili, served with collard greens.

Wednesday

Breakfast: Fresh-pressed apple juice and slow-cooked oatmeal with dates, raisins, walnuts, and bananas.

Lunch: Grilled soy cheese with tomato and a small side salad.

Dinner: Shepherd's pie with vegan mashed potatoes, fake ground meat, lentils, corn, and sautèed spinach and mushrooms.

Thursday

Breakfast: Fresh-squeezed OJ, an entire grapefruit, and a whole grain muffin.

Lunch: Veggie chili with an avocado-tomato salad and a handful of baked corn chips.

Dinner: Fusilli with zucchini, olives, basil, tomato, garlic, and olive oil served with whole grain Italian bread.

Friday

Breakfast: Fresh-squeezed OJ and cereal with peaches, banana, blackberries, and soymilk.

Lunch: Cucumber and avocado roll with miso soup and a small salad.

Dinner: No-cheese or vegan-cheese pizza loaded with veggies!

Saturday

Breakfast: Fake egg sandwich.

Lunch: Fake chicken Caesar salad.

Dinner: Steamed cauliflower, broccoli, carrots, and red cabbage over brown rice.

Sunday

Breakfast: Create your own fruit smoothie!

Lunch: Veggie burger with sautèed mushrooms, avocado, lettuce, tomato, onion, and sprouts served with roasted potato wedges.

Dinner: Fake chicken patty with BBQ sauce, black-eyed peas, collard greens, and corn on the cob.

*Feel free to snack on a handful of raw organic nuts each day.

**If you really want to treat yourself right, have fresh-pressed veggie juice every day. (Fresh-pressed, not packaged or pasteurized.)

***Don't forget to include organic, caffeine-free teas and to drink eight glasses of water a day.

****We include a list of recommended cookbooks toward the end of the book. Either buy a book or use the Internet for easy vegan recipes. One great site, veganpeace.com, includes recipes and a review of veggie cookbooks. Another winner is VegCooking.com.

Feeling gutsy and wanna branch out on your own? Go for it—shop 'till you drop. Here are ingredient lists of unfamiliar terms to help with your grocery outings. (Please be warned, this section is boring.)

Bad or Potentially
Bad Ingredients*

Alanine or amino acids: The building blocks of protein in all animals and plants. Make sure they are plant derived.

Albumen or albumin: Found in eggs, milk, muscles, blood, and many vegetable tissues and fluids. May cause allergic reaction. In cakes, cookies, candies, and some wines.

Ambergris: From whale intestines. Used as a flavoring in foods and beverages.

Aminosuccinate Acid or **aspartic acid:** Can be animal or plant source (e.g., molasses).

Arachidyl proprionate: A wax that can be from animal fat. Alternatives are peanut or vegetable oil.

Artificial Color, FD & C food color: Derived from coal-tar. Can contain trace amounts of lead and arsenic. Potentially carcinogenic. Alternatives: coloring from grapes, beets, turmeric, saffron, carrots, chlorophyll, annatto, alkanet.

Beta carotene, provitamin A: A pigment found in many animal tissues and in all plants. Used in the manufacturing of

Vitamin A. Make sure it is derived from plant sources.

Bone meal: Crushed or ground animal bones. In some vitamins and supplements as a source of calcium.

Butylated Hhydroxyanisole (BHA), butylated hydroxytoluene (BHT): An antioxidant and/or preservative commonly found in baked goods, canned items, powdered soups, bacon, foods containing artificial colors or flavors. Can cause cancer, birth defects, and infertility.

Carmine, cochineal, carminic acid: Red pigment from the crushed female cochineal insect. Reportedly, 70,000 beetles must be killed to produce one pound of this red dye. Used in red applesauce, and other foods (including red lollipops and food coloring). May cause allergic reaction.

Casein, caseinate, sodium caseinate: Milk protein found in dairy products, as well as "non-dairy" creamers, and soy cheese.

Cysteine, L-form: An amino acid from hair, which can come from animals. Used in some bakery products.

Cystine: An amino acid found in urine and horsehair. Used as a nutritional supplement.

Duodenum substances: From the digestive tracts of cows and pigs.

Added to some vitamin tablets.

Fatty acids: Can be one or any mixture of liquid and solid acids
such as caprylic, lauric, myristic, oleic, palmitic, and stearic.
Alternatives: vegetable-derived acids, soy lecithin.

Fish liver oil: Used in vitamins, supplements, and milk fortified
with vitamin D. Alternative: yeast extract ergosterol.

Gelatin, gel: Protein obtained by boiling skin, tendons, ligaments,
and/or bones with water. From cows and pigs. Used as a
thickener for fruit gelatins and puddings and in vitamins as a
coating and as capsules. In candies, marshmallows, cakes, ice
cream, yogurts. Sometimes used to assist in "clearing" wines.
Alternatives: carrageen (carrageenan, Irish moss), seaweeds
(algin, agar-agar, kelp), pectin from fruits, dextrins, locust
bean gum, cotton gum.

Glycerin, glycerol: A byproduct of soap manufacturing (normally
uses animal fat). In foods, mouthwashes, chewing gum,
toothpastes. Derivatives: Glycerides, Glyceryls,
Glycrethglycreth-26, Polyglycerol. Alternatives: vegetable
glycerin—a byproduct of vegetable oil soap, derivatives of
seaweed.

Isinglass: A form of gelatin prepared from the internal membranes of fish bladders. Sometimes used in "clearing" wines and in foods. Alternatives: bentonite clay, "Japanese isinglass," agar-agar. (See alternatives to Gelatin).

Lactic acid: Found in blood and muscle tissue. Also in sour milk, beer, sauerkraut, pickles, and other food products made by bacterial fermentation. Alternative: lactic acid from beets, plant-milk sugars.

Lactose: Milk sugar from milk of mammals. In foods, tablets, baked goods. Alternatives: plant-milk sugars.

Lard: Fat from hog abdomens. In baked goods, French fries, refried beans. Alternatives: pure vegetable fats or oils.

Lecithin or choline bitartrate: Waxy substance in nervous tissue of all living organisms, but frequently obtained for commercial purposes from eggs and soybeans. Also from blood or milk. Alternatives: soybean lecithin or corn-derived.

Lipase: Enzyme from the stomachs and tongue glands of calves, baby goats, and lambs. Used in cheese-making and in digestive aids. Alternatives: vegetable enzymes, castor beans.

Lipoids, lipids: Fat and fat-like substances that are found in animals and plants. Alternatives: vegetable oils.

Marine oil: From fish or marine mammals (including porpoises). Used as a shortening, especially in some margarines. Alternatives: vegetable oils.

Methionine: Essential amino acid found in various proteins (usually from egg albumen and casein). Used for freshness in potato chips.

Monoglycerides, glycerides, (See Glycerin): From animal fat. In margarines, cake mixes, candies, foods, etc. Alternative: vegetable glycerides.

Monosodium glutamate (MSG): Flavor enhancer blamed for reproductive, nervous system, and brain disorders. Found in soups, sauces, gravies, and sometimes hidden in baby food, baby formula, low-fat and no-fat milk, candy, gum, processed foods, and applied to non-organic fruits and vegetables as a wax or pesticide.

Myristal, ether sulfate, myristic acid: Organic acid in most animal and vegetable fats. In butter acids and food flavorings. Derivatives: isopropyl myristate, myristal ether sulfate, myristyls, oleyl myristate. Alternatives: nut butters, oil of lovage, coconut oil, extract from seed kernels of nutmeg, etc.

"Natural sources": Can mean animal or vegetable sources. Most often in the health food industry (especially in the cosmetics area), it means animal sources, such as animal elastin, glands, fat, protein, and oil. Alternatives: plant sources.

Nitrates: Potentially deadly, carcinogenic preservatives. Found in processed foods and meats.

Nucleic acids: In the nucleus of all living cells. Used in vitamins, supplements. Alternatives: plant sources.

Oleic acid: Obtained from various animal and vegetable fats and oils. Usually obtained commercially from inedible tallow. (See Tallow.) Alternatives: coconut oil.

Olestra: A fat substitute found in low fat and dairy-type products that reduces fat-soluble vitamins in the body.

Panthenol, dexpanthenol, vitamin B-Complex complex factor, provitamin B-5: Can come from animal, plant, or synthetic sources, so be sure to buy only plant-based.

Pepsin: In hogs' stomachs. A clotting agent. In some cheeses and vitamins. Same uses and alternatives as Rennet. (see Rennet)

Polysorbates: Derivatives of fatty acids.

Potassium bisulfite, sodium bisulfite, sulfur dioxide: Used as anti-fungal, anti-browning, or antioxidant in cheeses, processed meats, canned fruits and vegetables, dried fruits, and/or baked goods. Can cause asthma, shock, or death.

Potassium bromate: Found in baked goods, can cause cancer and kidney and nervous system disorders. Banned worldwide except Japan and U.S.

Rapeseed Oil: An emulsifier and stabilizer found in baked goods, dairy products, processed meats. Can cause cancer, heart disease, vision loss.

Rennet, rennin: Enzyme from calves' stomachs. Used in cheese-making and in many coagulated dairy products. Alternatives: lemon juice or vegetable rennet.

Saccharine: Artificial sweetener found to cause cancer.

Stearic acid: Fat from cows and sheep and from dogs and cats euthanized in animal shelters, etc. Most often refers to a fatty substance taken from the stomachs of pigs. Used in gum, food flavoring. Derivatives: stearamide, stearamine, stearates, stearic hydrazide, stearone, stearoxytrimethylsilane, stearoyl lactylic acid, stearyl betaine, stearyl imidazoline. Alternatives: Stearic acid can be found in many vegetable fats, coconut.

Tallow, fatty alcohol: Rendered beef fat. May cause eczema and blackheads.

Urea, uric acid, carbamide: Excreted from urine and other bodily fluids. Used to "brown" baked goods, such as pretzels. Derivatives: imidazolidinyl urea, uric acid.

Vitamin A: Can come from fish liver oil (e.g., shark liver oil), egg yolk, butter, and synthetics. In vitamins, supplements. Alternatives: carrots, other vegetables, lemongrass, wheat germ oil.

Vitamin B-12: Can come from animal products or bacteria cultures. Alternatives: Vegetarian vitamins, fortified soymilks, nutritional yeast, fortified faux meat substitutes. Vitamin B-12 is often listed as "cyanocobalamin" on food labels. Vegan health professionals caution that vegans get 5-10 mcg/day of vitamin B-12 from fortified foods or supplements .

Vitamin D, ergocalciferol, vitamin D-2, ergosterol, provitamin D-2, calciferol, vitamin D-3: Vitamin D can come from fish liver oil, milk, egg yolk, etc. Vitamin D-2 can come from animal

fats or plant sterols. Vitamin D-3 is always from an animal
source. Alternatives: plant and mineral sources, completely
vegetarian vitamins, exposure of skin to sunlight.

Whey: A derivative of milk. Usually in cakes, cookies, candies, and
breads. Used in cheese-making. Alternatives: soybean whey.

Bear in mind, even though these are on our "bad" list, they are fine
when derived from non-chemical, non-animal sources.

Scary-Sounding But Actually Harmless Ingredients*

Alpha tocopherol, Alpha tocopherol acetate: Vitamin E derived
from corn, peanuts, or soy.

Arrowroot: A natural thickening starch, derived from the arrowroot plant.

Absorbic acid: Synthetic vitamin C, often derived from corn.

Brown rice syrup: A sweetener derived from brown rice.

Cellulose: Plant fiber.

Coconut Oil: Great for frying and baking because it can withstand
high heats without becoming carcinogenic. Also helps the

body metabolize fatty acids.

Date Sugar: Sweetener derived from dates.

Inulin: Present in many herbs. Acts as a probiotic and promotes healthy intestinal tract.

Linoleic acid: Derived from corn, soy, or peanuts.

Saffron: Natural food coloring derived from a plant.

Sucanat: SUgar CAne NATural, a natural sweetener.

*Sourced from *Food Additives: A Shopper's Guide To What's Safe & What's Not* by Christine Hoza Farlow, D.C., and PETA's *Caring Consumer Guide.*[220]

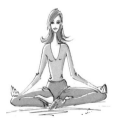

Chapter 12

FYI

U m, just bcause we wrote this book doesn't mean we're perfect. If you see us eating junk food or doing beer bongs, don't hold it against us. We believe in enjoying life *and* maintaining a healthy balance. We're human. Also, we have some fat, gross body parts, too. We're women.

❧

Yeah, eating onions and garlic makes your breath smell like someone took a shit down your throat. But they fight cancer and help detoxify your liver. So eat 'em.

What's all the drama surrounding hydrogenated oils? We'll tell you. Manufacturers add hydrogen to mono- or polyunsaturated fats (good fats), in order to change their consistencies. The end result, trans-fatty acids (bad), is a more solid product with a longer shelf life. Margarines, cookies, cakes, doughnuts, potato chips, meat and dairy products, and shortening can all contain hydrogenated oils. Trans-fatty acids can cause derangements of cell structure, accelerated aging, and a predisposition to diseases.[221]

Think about it. They are literally altering a naturally occurring product's molecular structure by adding hydrogen molecules to it. Eating these chemically altered foods containing hydrogenated oils will increase your risk of heart disease. Sad to say, heating oil at high temperatures also changes its natural molecular configuration and produces free-radicals. Free-radicals not only destroy essential fats and vitamins but are also linked to cancer and heart disease.[222] This is why olive oil and peanut oil, which are both healthy, can be very *unhealthy* in dishes like fried eggplant or

French fries. Avoid eating fried foods (sniffle) and re-using heated oils. Never heat oil to the point where it is smoking. Cook with canola oil or coconut oil using low heat and for the shortest amount of time possible.

❧

Don't be a cheap asshole. Yeah, yeah, yeah, organic produce is usually more expensive than conventional produce. But we spend countless dollars on clothes, jewelry, manicures, magazines, rent or mortgages, car payments, and other bullshit. Surely our health and our bodies (we only get one body) are more important than anything else in our lives. Even if you are spending more on organic food, you'll save money in the long run if you're preparing more meals and snacks at home (which is always cheaper than buying food on the fly). Organic is worth the extra money, and you should aim to have everything you eat be organic. But especially when buying fruits or vegetables that you eat without peeling the skin. Always buy organic blueberries, strawberries, raspberries, apples, and pears. Peanuts and peanut butter, too, because conventional ones are loaded with pesticides. Buying organic produce is the only way to guarantee you're not eating genetically modified organisms. According to *Food Additives: A Shopper's Guide to What's Safe & What's Not,* "genes are taken from one species of plant, animal or virus and inserted into another species in order to produce a desirable trait, such as disease resistance or hardier crops. No one knows the long-term effects of eating genetically modified foods. Genetically modified foods are being sold now and they are not being labeled. Certified organic foods are the only foods guaranteed not to be genetically modified."[223]

Brushing your teeth is a great way to ward off sweet cravings and stop yourself from eating. But, two or three times a day, every day for your entire life, you swallow trace amounts of toothpaste. What's in it? Chemicals? Artificial sweeteners? Would you eat it? Read the ingredients. Buy natural.

The skin is the body's largest organ. Every day, we slop all sorts of potions and lotions and makeup on ourselves, and rub them into our skin. Ever read the ingredients of these products? Ever consider that you are putting chemicals directly onto your largest organ? Ever think about the pores all over your body and what you're putting inside them? Hopefully, you will now. Buy natural beauty products. What you put *on* your body is just as important as what you put *in* your body (because, in essence, what you put on your body will wind up in your body), especially on body parts you shave, pluck, or wax. Open pores do not want chemicals bulldozing through. Are your deodorant, makeup, perfumes, and lotions safe?

❧

You can get too much of a good thing. So don't overdose on water, or you'll flush necessary salt supplies right out of your body. Eight glasses a day is a good target.

❧

Natural, unrefined Celtic sea salt (different from table salt) contains many essential minerals, enhances organ function, and neutralizes toxins. It also contributes to the hydration of our cells and organs.[224]

❧

Buy a food steamer. It will change your life.

❧

Do yoga. It is a kick-ass cardio workout that will strengthen, tone, and harden your muscles. Yoga is amazing for organ function, immune system strength, tackling insomnia, improving PMS symptoms and menstrual cramps, and overall health. You will love how it makes you look and feel. All kidding aside, if everyone did yoga, we would have world peace.

❧

Donate blood. You can save a life and lose weight at the same time.

❧

Keep your eyes peeled for bad press regarding veganism. It's usually planted by the industries that are threatened by the movement. Don't believe any of it. It's all bogus bullshit. One study claimed that feeding children a vegan diet was tantamount to child abuse. It just so happens that the National Cattlemen's Beef Association paid for the study. They had the gall to experiment on African children who were literally starving. These children were eating nothing but corn and beans in minuscule servings. When servings of meat were added to their diets, their health improved.[225] Well, of course it did. They were fucking starving. This doesn't prove that veganism is dangerous or unhealthy. It just shows that the National Cattlemen's Beef Association will exploit starving, impoverished children to create bad press for veganism and boost its own meat sales. This is nothing short of a disgrace and an embarrassment to America.

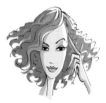

Chapter 13

Use Your Head

on't be a fat pig anymore. You know what you have to do, now do it. But don't go anorexic on us, either. It's easy to get caught up in any lifestyle change and go overboard. Make healthy choices and take excellent care of yourself without getting neurotic and obsessive.

USE YOUR HEAD. We can't say it enough. Use your own head and think about what you are eating. Forget what you've ever read, heard, or learned and just think for yourself. Once they've recovered, your body, brain, and instincts will always lead you down the right food path. Obey them and disregard everyone and everything else. You know the truth.

Read the ingredients. This goes hand in hand with using your head. If you plan on eating something, you should know exactly what it is. Even if it's a product that we've recommended, you still need to check the ingredients. Companies change their recipes all the time. Two vegan products we loved initially and suggested weren't vegan by the time we were finished writing this book, and we had to remove them from our recommendation lists. Trust no one. Not even us. Some of the products on our suggested food lists aren't perfect; we make certain allowances based on our own opinions and desires. Read and decide for yourself. And if you don't recognize an ingredient, call the company's 800 number on the package and ask what it is. If it's not something you would put in your body, tell them, and suggest that they improve their product. Companies really do take comments into account, so always voice your opinion.

Now that you're a Skinny Bitch, don't turn into a skinny bitch. We conceived of the title, *Skinny Bitch*, to get attention and sell books. We just wanted to spread our message far and wide and thought *Skinny Bitch* was a good way to do it. But we are not bitches, and we have no desire to promote bitchiness. There is nothing uglier than a pretty woman who's nasty. If you look great, you should feel good about yourself and be happy. Instead of fixating on the last five pounds you want to lose, celebrate the five you already lost. Progress, not perfection. Don't be insecure or competitive or feel threatened by women who are thinner or prettier than you. Be happy for them; it will make you look better. Smile a lot, give compliments out whenever you can, and be nice to everyone. You'll just keep getting prettier and prettier and skinnier and skinnier.

Soon, you'll notice people (especially men) flocking to the new you. Not just because you're skinny but because you are happier, healthier, and eating a cruelty-free diet. So feel free to share your new wealth of information with everyone who asks. Spread the good word, but be careful not to preach. You'll see that some people get very defensive about their diets when you tell them about yours. Even if you are being very non-judgmental, people may feel threatened by your righteousness. Understandably, your being a vegan shines a spotlight on the cruelty they're contributing to, and it makes them feel uncomfortable. When asked, you can describe what you've learned about the treatment of farm animals and all of the health benefits of being vegan. By all means, let people know how great you feel and how much weight you've lost. But never suggest that they try it or make them feel bad about their diet. Offer to lend them your copy of *Skinny Bitch*, or give them the GoVeg.com website. But don't push it. Everyone seeks the truth in his or her own time.

Now that you've got your diet, health, and appearances under control, fix other areas of your life. After all, there's no point in being gorgeous if your life is a mess. End your co-dependent relationship, quit your dead-end job, and ditch your toxic friends. Make a list of goals and start chipping away at them. THIS IS YOUR LIFE! Live it to the fullest with reckless abandon. Seize the day. And do it again tomorrow. Live. Go get your dream job. Search for your dream man. Fear nothing. Try everything. Be excited. Dance. You'll never get yesterday back, but today is yours for the taking. Make it great.

Bravo. You've got your life and your diet on-track. But you still need to move your ass. Exercise will boost your self-esteem, reduce your junk-food cravings, and help you *lose weight*. If you can commit to a gym routine, fantastic! You will reach your fitness goals faster. But you don't need to be a gym rat. Just do something! It can even be fun. Take a class that you've always wondered about, like kickboxing or belly dancing. Go for walks after dinner or bike rides on weekends. Better yet, walk or bike to work. Whatever you choose, exercise makes you feel great about yourself. And that alone is priceless.

You *are* what you *think*. Our thoughts, feelings, beliefs, and experiences create tangible, concrete reactions at cellular and atomic levels. So whether something is "real" or not doesn't matter. If we think, feel, believe, or experience it, it will become a reality. Slow down and think about this and realize the implications it can have on your life. It can work for or against you. For example, if you *think* you are fat and that diets never work and that you'll always be fat, then yes, you *are* fat and diets never work and you will always be fat. What you *think* actually becomes embedded in your brain and your cells and the energy field surrounding you. Your thoughts are just that powerful. So if you *feel* you are meant to be thin, and *believe Skinny Bitch* will make you lose weight and *know* that this book is going to change your life, you *will* be thin, you *will* lose weight, and your life *will* change. It is just that simple.

In her book, *Anatomy of the Spirit*, Dr. Caroline Myss examines the unquestionable link between negative emotions and physical illnesses. Take "Julie," for example. Julie's husband treated her with contempt and disdain, frequently said the mere sight of her repulsed him, and refused to sleep with her. It is no coincidence that Julie was diagnosed with breast and ovarian cancer, reflecting her lack of self-love for her "womanhood." She could not leave her husband. She never recovered from her cancer and died as a result.[226] "Joanna" was married to a man who had multiple affairs, which she knew about but tried to live with. Not surprisingly, she developed breast cancer. Eventually, she confronted her husband and demanded fidelity. However, he was unable to change, so she left the marriage. Joanna recovered from her cancer. *Anatomy of the Spirit* chronicles one history after another of people sickening themselves or healing themselves with thought and emotion. (Of course, we are not suggesting that everyone suffering from a disease has brought it upon him or herself. We are, however, saying it is entirely possible to do so.)

Our minds are infinitely powerful. Our favorite self-help gurus, Dr. Wayne Dyer, Louise Hay, and Tony Robbins, understand this, and they all preach the power of daily affirmations. An affirmation is a positive statement you make that allows you to clearly envision a goal or mindset. It is declared as if it is already happening, and it can be anything you want:

"Every day in every way my ass is getting smaller."

"Every day in every way my thighs are getting thinner."

"Every day in every way my stomach is getting flatter."

"Every day in every way I'm losing more and more weight."

"Every day in every way I'm loving my body more."

"Every day in every way I'm getting healthier and healthier."

Create your own affirmations and say them (in your head or aloud, if you can) when you wake up in the morning, while exercising, in your car, and in bed at night. You will immediately notice how good they make you feel and you will be astonished at the results. This book is the result of our affirmations, so we *know* they truly work.

Now that you love yourself, wear sexy clothes. You worked hard for this body and you should be proud of it. We know it can be terrifying to wear something super-trendy—like you don't have the right or aren't worthy. But you *are* good enough, you *do* deserve it, and no one is thinking otherwise. So don't be afraid of wearing revealing, high-fashion clothes. This is your body for this lifetime. Dress it up and love it. Why are you "saving" all your good underwear or hot outfits? Wear them, fool. But please keep in mind that looking cheap or cheesy doesn't accomplish anything. If you have poor fashion sense (you know who you are), ask someone for guidance.

Now we know we keep encouraging you to look your best, but, for the love of God, don't associate your worth with your appearance. We are spiritual beings walking around in these crazy skin suits. Our insides are much more important than our outsides. So don't you fucking dare measure your worth by the amount of attention or validation you get from men. It's nice to be appreciated, but it is not a necessity. Love yourself and your looks, even if no one else seems to. In time, your confidence and self-love will attract a winner.

Well, it's all there in black and white. We sincerely hope you will take the knowledge you've learned and put it to use from this moment on. YOU hold the power to change your life, and it's really so simple. Use your head, lose your ass.

Afterword

Isn't man an amazing animal? He kills wildlife by the millions in order to protect his domestic animals and their feed. Then he kills domestic animals by the billions and eats them. This in turn kills man by the millions, because eating all those animals leads to degenerative—and fatal—health conditions like heart disease, kidney disease, and cancer. So then man tortures and kills millions more animals to look for cures for these diseases. Elsewhere, millions of other human beings are being killed by hunger and malnutrition because food they could eat is being used to fatten domestic animals. Meanwhile, some people are dying of sad laughter at the absurdity of man, who kills so easily and so violently, and once a year sends out cards praying for "Peace on Earth."

—Preface from *Old MacDonald's Factory Farm,*
by C. David Coates

Recommended Reading

Books

Slaughterhouse, Gail A. Eisnitz. *This book is an absolute *must-read* for every American who has ever eaten meat, is still considering eating meat, or isn't sure if they should or shouldn't. Buy this book today!

Vegan: The New Ethics of Eating, Erik Marcus

The Food Revolution, John Robbins

Fast Food Nation, Eric Schlosser

Breaking the Food Seduction, Neal Barnard, M.D.

Carbophobia: The Sorry Truth About America's Low-Carb Craze, Michael Greger, M.D.

A Way Out: Dis-ease Deception & The Truth About Health, Matthew Grace (matthewgrace.com)

Magazines

VegNews (vegnews.com)   *Satya* (satyamag.com)

Spiritual/Self-Help Books/CDs

Your Erroneous Zones, Dr. Wayne Dyer

Real Magic, Dr. Wayne Dyer

You'll See It When You Believe It, Dr. Wayne Dyer

Notes from a Friend, Anthony Robbins

Get the Edge CDs, Anthony Robbins

You Can Heal Your Life, Louise L. Hay

Anatomy of the Spirit, Caroline Myss, Ph.D.

Cookbooks

The Uncheese Cookbook, Joanne Stepaniak

The Garden of Vegan, Tanya Barnard and Sara Kramer

How it all Vegan, by Tanya Barnard and Sara Kramer

The Compassionate Cook, PETA & Ingrid Newkirk

CalciYum, David & Rachelle Bronfman

The Native Foods Restaurant Cookbook, Tanya Petrovna

The Candle Cafè Cookbook, Joy Pierson and Bart Potenza with
Barbara Scott-Goodman

Viva le Vegan!, Dreena Burton

Very Vegetarian, Jannequin Bennet

Veganpeace.com offers recipes and reviews of veggie cookbooks

Restaurant Guides

vegoutguide.com

happycow.net

vegdining.com

The Tofu Tollbooth, Elizabeth Zipern and Dar Williams

VegOut: Vegetarian Dining Guide to New York City,
      Justin Schwartz

VegOut: Vegetarian Dining Guide to Seattle and Portland,
      George B. Stevenson

VegOut: Vegetarian Dining Guide to Washington, D.C.,
      Andrew Evans

VegOut: Vegetarian Dining Guide to San Francisco,
      Michele Ana Jordan

VegOut: Vegetarian Dining Guide to Southern California,
      Kathy Lynn Siegel

VegOut: Vegetarian Dining Guide to Chicago,
    Margaret Littman

VegOut: Vegetarian Dining Guide to Houston,
    Ann Sieber

VegOut: Vegetarian Dining Guide to Salt Lake City/Denver,
    Andrea Mather

Merchandise
Web Sites

veganstore.com

VeganEssentials.com

AnimalRights Stuff.com

AlternativeOutfitters.com

feelgoodtees.com

mooshoes.com

veganunlimited.com

TheVegetarianSite.com

VegSexShop.com

Web Sites

skinnybitch.net

GoVeg.com

meat.org

peta.org

farmsanctuary.org

pcrm.org

cok.net

protectinganimals.org

veganmd.org

atkinsexposed.org

VeganOutreach.org

afa-online.org

informedeating.org

organicconsumers.org

holisticmed.com

congress.org

anthonyrobbinsdc.com

drwaynedyer.com

hayhouse.com

oa.org (overeaters anonymous), 505-891-2664

Food Web Sites

vegieworld.com

deliciouschoices.com

veganstore.com

rawbalance.com

playfood.org

TreeHugginTreats.com

simpletreats.com

chocolatedecadence.com

leaheyfoods.com

vegandreams.com

goodbaker.com

rosecitychocolates.com

eatraw.com

nutrilicious.com

allisonsgourmet.com

healthy-eating.com

Sources Consulted

Armstrong, Clare, MS, RD. DiscoveryHealth.com. The Discovery Channel, updated Sept. 25, 2002; accessed Jan. 20, 2005

http://health.discovery.com/encyclopedias/1940.html

Aspartame Victims Support Group, presidiotex.com, updated Jan. 13, 2005; accessed Jan. 20, 2005, http://www.presidiotex.com/aspartame/

Atkins, Robert C., M.D. *Dr. Atkins' New Diet Revolution.* New York: Avon, 2002.

Baillie-Hamilton, Paula, M.D., Ph.D. *The Body Restoration Plan.* New York: Avery, 2003.

"Banned as Human Food, StarLink Corn Found in Food Aid." *Environmental News Service,* Feb. 16, 2005; accessed Feb. 20, 2005, http://www.ens-newswire.com/ens/feb2005/2005-02-16-09.asp#anchor2

"Barcelona Report," presidiotex.com, Jan. 12, 2005, accessed Sept. 9, 2005, http://www.presidiotex.com/barcelona/

Barnard, Neal M.D. *Breaking The Food Seduction: The Hidden Reasons Behind Food Cravings—and 7 Steps to End Them Naturally.* New York: St. Martin's, 2003.

Beck, Leslie, R.D. *The Ultimate Nutrition Guide For Women: How to Stay Healthy with Diet, Vitamins, Minerals, and Herbs.* Hoboken: John Wiley & Sons, 2001.

Bellon, Roberta. National Justice League. "Aspartame Lawsuits Accuse Many Companies Of Poisoning The Public," April 6, 2004, accessed Feb. 10, 2005, http://www.newmedia-explorer.org/sepp/2004/04/09/aspartame_neurotoxic_coca_cola_pepsi_nutra_sweet_sued_in_california.htm

Boschen, Hank. "Cycles of the Body," thejuiceguy.com, Feb. 10, 2005, http://www.juiceguy.com/cycle.shtml

Bray, George A., Samara Joy Nielson, and Barry M. Popkin. "Consumption of high-fructose corn syrup in beverages may play a role in the epidemic of obesity." *American Journal of Clinical Nutrition,* Vol. 79, No. 4, 537-543, April 2004, http://www.ajcn.org/cgi/content/abstract/79/4/537. 1 From the Pennington Biomedical Research Center, Louisiana State University, Baton Rouge, LA (GAB), and the Department of Nutrition, University of North Carolina, Chapel Hill (SJN and BMP).

Brown, Harold. e-mail to Rory Freedman, March 21, 2005.

Brownlee, Christen. *The Beef about UTIs,* Vol. 167 no. 3, Jan. 15, 2005; accessed Jan. 20, 2005, http://www.sciencenews.org/articles/20050115/food.asp

Burros, Marian. "Splenda's 'Sugar' Claim Unites Odd Couple of Nutrition Wars." *New York Times,* Feb. 15, 2005; accessed Feb. 20, 2005, www.skyhen.org/CorporatePower/splendas_sugar_claim_unites_odd_couple_of_nutrition_wars.php

Caffeine. eCureMe Inc., accessed Feb. 10, 2005,

http://life.ecureme.com/healthyliving/naturalmedicine/n_caffeine.asp

Caring Consumer Guide. Peta.org, accessed March 26, 2005,
www.caringconsumer.com/ingredientslist.html

Chandel, Amar. "Sweet Poison," *The Tribune Spectrum,* March 14,
2004; accessed March 22, 2005, www.tribuneindia.com/2004/
20040314/spectrum/main1.htm

Cichoke, Anthony J., D.C. *Enzymes & Enzyme Therapy: How to
Jump Start Your Way to Lifelong Good Health.* New Canaan:
Keats Publishing Inc., 1994.

Coates, C. David. *Old MacDonald's Factory Farm.* New York: The
Continuum Publishing Co., 1989.

Cohen, Robert. *Essence of Betrayal,* accessed March 1, 2005,
http://www.notmilk.com/forum/594.html

"Common Dairy Digestive Under-Recognized and Under-
Diagnosed in Minorities." Johnson & Johnson, accessed Feb.
13, 2005, ww.jnj.com/news/jnj_news/20020311_0944.htm

Cook, Christopher D. "Environmental Hogwash: The EPA works
with factory farms to delay regulation of 'Extremely
Hazardous Substances.' " Oct. 6, 2004; accessed Jan. 27,
2005, www.inthesetimes.com/site/main/print/environmen-
tal_hogwash/

Cousens, Gabriel M.D. *Conscious Eating.* Berkeley: North Atlantic
Books, 2000.

Cousin, Jean Pierre and Kirsten Hartvig. *Vitality Foods For Health and Fitness.* London: Duncan Baird, 2002.

Davis, Gail. "A Tale of Two Sweeteners: Aspartame & Stevia," accessed Feb. 12, 2005, http://suewidemark.netfirms.com/davis.htm

Des Maisons, Kathleen, Ph.D. *Potatoes Not Prozac.* New York: Fireside, 1998.

Diamond, Harvey and Marilyn. *Fit For Life.* New York: Warner, 1985.

Diamond, Harvey and Marilyn. *Fit For Life II: Living Health.* New York: Warner, 1987.

Eisnitz, Gail A. 'Ask the Experts.' Peta.org, accessed March 17, 2005, www.goveg.com/vegkit/meet.asp

Eisnitz, Gail A. *Slaughterhouse: The Shocking Story of Greed, Neglect, and Inhumane Treatment Inside the U.S. Meat Industry*. Amherst: Prometheus Books, 1997.

"Factory Farming: Environmental Consequences." Animalalliance.ca, accessed March 29, 2005, www.animalalliance.ca/kids/facfar1.htm#environment

"Fact vs. Fiction." Thetruthaboutsplenda.com, accessed Feb. 14, 2005, www.truthaboutsplenda.com/factvsfiction/index.html

Farlow, Christine Hoza, D.C. *Food Additives: A Shopper's Guide to What's Safe & What's Not*. Escondido: KISS for Health, 2004.

"FDA Approved Animal Drug Products." FDA 'Green Book'

section, accessed March 21, 2005,
http://dil.vetmed.vt.edu/NadaFirst/ NADA.cfm

"Fish and Shellfish: Contamination Problems Preclude Inclusion in the Dietary Guidelines for Americans." Pcrm.org, Spring 2004, accessed March 31, 2005, www.pcrm.org/health/reports/ fish_report.html

"Fish Feel Pain." Fishinghurts.com, accessed March 3, 2005, www.fishinghurts.com/FishFeelPain.asp

"Food Additives." New-fitness.com, accessed Feb. 4, 2005, www.new-fitness.com/nutrition/food_additives.html

"Food and Nutrition Assistance Programs." Economic Research Service, U.S. Department of Agriculture, USDA.gov; updated March 18, 2005; accessed March 22, 2005, www.ers.usda.gov/Briefing/FoodNutritionAssistance/

"Free-Range Eggs and Meat: Conning Consumers?" Peta.org, accessed March 16, 2005, http://www.peta.org/mc/factsheet_display.asp?ID=96

Fuhrman, Joel M.D. *Eat to Live*. Boston, New York, London: Little, Brown, 2003.

Gates, Donna. *The Body Ecology Diet.* (excerpt from), accessed Feb. 25, 2005, http://www.holisticmed.com/sweet/stv-cook.txt

Gee, Margaret. *Words of Wisdom Calendar*. Kansas City, MI: Andrews McMeel, 2004.

Gold, Mark. "Formaldehyde Poisoning from Aspartame," Dec. 9,

1998; accessed March 6, 2005, www.holisticmed.com/aspar-
tame/embalm.html

Gold, Mark. "Aspartame/NutraSweet Toxicity Summary" Nov. 30,
2000; accessed March 3, 2005, www.holisticmed.com/aspar-
tame/summary.html

Gold, Mark. "Common Toxic and Unhealthy Substances to Avoid,"
accessed Feb. 28, 2005, http://www.holisticmed.com/aspar-
tame/history.faq

Gold, Mark. "Scientific Abuse in Methanol/Formaldehyde
Research Related to Aspartame," accessed Jan. 12, 2005,
http://www.holisticmed.com/aspartame/abuse/methanol.html

Gold, Mark. "Toxicity Effects of Aspartame Use," accessed Feb. 2,
2005, www.holisticmed.com/aspartame/

Gold, Mark D. "The Bitter Truth about Artificial Sweeteners."
truthcampaign.ukf.net. accessed March 23, 2005,
http://www.truthcampaign.ukf.net/ articles/health/aspar-
tame.html

Grace, Matthew. *A Way Out: Dis-Ease Deception and The Truth
About Health.* U.S.A: Matthew Grace, 2000.

"The Great Sugar Debate: Is It Vegan?" accessed Feb. 20, 2005,
http://www.vegfamily.com/articles/sugar.htm

Greger, Michael, M.D. "Rocket Fuel in Milk," accessed Jan. 23,
2005, http://all-creatures.org/health/rocket.html

Green, Che. "Not Milk: The USDA, Monsanto, and the U.S. Dairy

Industry." *LiP Magazine,* July 9, 2002; accessed Feb. 20, 2005, http://www.alternet.org/story/13557/

Grogan, Bryanna Clark. "A Few Words About Sugar and Other Sweeteners," accessed Feb. 22, 2005, http://www.vegsource.com/articles/bryanna_sugar.htm

"Growing and Processing Sugar." The Sugar Association; accessed Jan. 12, 2005, http://www.sugar.org/facts/grow.html

Harris, Simon. "Organic Consumers Association (OCA) Denounces Degradation of Organic Food Standards by Congress,"accessed Feb. 10, 2005, http://environment.about.com/ library/pressrelease/bloca.htm

Hasselberger, Sepp. "Aspartame: RICO Complaint Filed Against NutraSweet, ADA, Monsanto." Sept. 17, 2004; accessed Feb. 15, 2005, http://www.newmediaexplorer.org/sepp/2004/09/17/ aspartame_rico_complaint_filed_against_nutrasweet_ada_m onsanto.htm

Hatherill, Robert J., Ph.D. *Eat to Beat Cancer.* Los Angeles: Renaissance Books, 1998.

Healthy Child Online Articles and Resources, accessed March 2, 2005, http://www.healthychild.com/database/life_is_sweet_ a_guide_to_using_healthy_sweeteners.htm

"The Hidden Lives of Chickens," accessed March 3, 2005, http://www.peta.org/feat/hiddenlives/

Holford, Patrick. *The Optimum Nutrition Bible.* Berkeley: The Crossing Press, 1999.

Howell, Edward M.D. *Enzyme Nutrition: The Food Enzyme Concept.* U.S.A.: Avery, 1985.

Howell, Laurie. "#193 Why Choose Organic Coffee?" accessed Feb. 25, 2005, http://www.thegreenscene.com/shows/193.html

"Investigation Reveals Slaughter Horrors at Agriprocessors." Peta.org, accessed March 17, 2005, www.goveg.com/feat/agriprocessors/

Johnson, Lucy. "Aspartame . . . A Killer!" *The Sunday Express* London, U.K. Newfrontier.com; accessed March 21, 2005, http://www.newfrontier.com/asheville/aspartame.htm

Kamen, Betty, Ph.D. *New Facts About Fiber.* Novato: Nutrition Encounter, 1991.

Krebs, A.V. "USDA Accused of Allowing 'Sham Certifiers' into the National Organic Program." *The Agribusiness Examiner.* Issue #367, Aug 23, 2004; accessed Jan 25, 2005; http://www.organicconsumers.org/organic/usda.cfm

Krumm, Susan. "Refining process has sweet ending." *Lawrence Journal-World,* June 13, 2001; accessed Jan. 20, 2005, http://ljworld.com/section/cookingqa/story/55875

Langeland, Terje. "Tainted Meat, Tainted Money: Consumer groups decry coziness between government, agribusiness." *Colorado Springs Independent online edition,* Aug. 1-7, 2002; accessed Feb. 20, 2005, http://www.csindy.com/csindy/2002-08-01/cover2.html

Langley, Gill, MA, Ph.D. *Vegan Nutrition: A Survey Of Research.*

Oxford: The Vegan Society, 1988.

"The Latest In Cancer: 'White Meat' Linked to Colon Cancer."
Pcrm.org, Winter 99; accessed March 28, 2005,
http://www.pcrm.org/magazine/GM99Winter9.html

Leake, Jonathon. "The rich and emotional lives of cows."
News.com; accessed Feb. 28, 2005, http://www.news.com/au/
story/0,10117,12390397-13762,00.html

Mason, Jim and Peter Singer. *Animal Factories*. New York: Crown,
1990.

McCaleb, Rob. "Stevia Leaf—Too Good To Be Legal?" Herb
Research Foundation, accessed Feb. 14, 2005,
http://www.holisticmed.com/sweet/stv-faq.txt

"Men's Health Warns of Foods You Should Never Eat." Peta.org,
accessed March 23, 2005, http://www.peta.org/feat/menshealth/

Mercola, Joseph, M.D. with Alison Rose Levy. *The No-Grain Diet:
Conquer Carbohydrate Addiction and Stay Slim for Life.* New
York: Dutton, 2003.

Mercola, Joseph, M.D. "The Potential Dangers of Sucralose."
vitaminlady.com; accessed Sept. 9, 2005, http://www.vitamin-
lady.com/articles/sucralose.asp

Mercola, Joseph, M.D. "The Secret Dangers of Splenda
(Sucralose), an Artificial Sweetener," Dec. 3, 2000; accessed
Feb. 20, 2005,
http://www.mercola.com/2000/dec/3/sucralose_dangers.htm

Mercola, Joseph, M.D. "Splenda—Here We Go Again." July 21, 2004; accessed Feb. 12, 2005, http://www.mercola.com/fcgi/pf/2004/jul/21/splenda.htm

Mercola, Joseph, M.D. "US 'Food Pyramid' Invalid as It was Made by Experts with Conflicts of Interest." Nov. 19, 2000; accessed Jan. 10, 2005, http://www.mercola.com/2000/nov/19/food_pyramid.htm

"Milk Sucks." Peta.org.; milksucks.com, accessed March 12, 2005, http://www.milksucks.com/

Mindell, Earl R., Ph.D. with Hester Mundis. *Earl Mindell's New Vitamin Bible.* New York, Boston: Warner, 2004.

"Molasses." Everything2com, Oct. 2, 2003; accessed Feb. 2, 2005, http://www.everything2.com/index.pl?node=molasses

"Molasses nutrition data." Nutritiondata.com, accessed March 3, 2005, http://www.nutritiondata.com/facts-001-02s04at.html

Murray, Rich. "How Aspartame Became Legal-The Timeline." Dec. 24, 2002; accessed March 5, 2005, http://www.quantumbalancing.com/news/aspartameap-proved.htm

Myss, Caroline, Ph.D. *Anatomy of the Spirit: The Seven Stages of Power and Healing.* New York: Three Rivers, 1996.

"National Cattleman's Beef Association Pays for Sadistic Anti-Vegan 'Study.'" Vegsource Interactive Inc., accessed Feb. 22, 2005, http://www.vegsource.com/articles2/ncbs_vegan_study.htm

"National Soft Drink Association Protest (Summary)"
    Congressional Record-Senate, March 11, 2005; accessed Jan.
    20, 2005, http://www.dorway.com/nsda.txt

"Nation's Largest Organic Dairy Brand, Horizon, Accused of
    Violating Organic Standards." The Cornucopia Institute,
    Feb. 16, 2005, accessed March 2, 2005, http://www.organic-
    consumers.org/organic/horizon21705.cfm

"Natural Sweeteners." Natural Nutrition, accessed Feb. 2, 2005,
    http://www.livrite.com/sweeten.htm

"Natural Sweetener-Safe for Diabetics," accessed Feb. 15, 2005,
    http://www.primalnature.com/stevia.html

Ness, Carol. "Organic Food: Outcry Over Rule Changes that Allow
    More Pesticides, Hormones." The San Francisco Chronicle,
    May 22, 2004, accessed March 2, 2005, http://www.common-
    dreams.org/cgi-bin/print.cgi?file=/headlines04/0522-09.htm

Nestle, Marion. *Food Politics: How the Food Industry Influences
    Nutrition and Health*. California: University of California,
    2000.

Notmilk.com. March 5, 2005, http://notmilk.com/forum/526.html

"OCA and Environmental Groups Sue USDA to Enforce Strict
    Standards: Environmental Groups Back Harvey Lawsuit."
    Organic Business News. December 2004, Vol. 16, no. 12;
    accessed Jan. 12, 2005,
    http://organicconsumers.org/organic/lawsuit010505.cfm

"Organic Industry and Consumers Celebrate USDA Reversal on

Non-Food National Organic Standards" press release, May 26, 2004; accessed Feb. 10, 2005, http://www.westonaprice.org/federalupdate/aa2004/infoalert_052604.html

Pert, Candace B., Ph.D. *Molecules of Emotion.* New York: Scribner, 1997

"Pigs: Smart Animals at the Mercy of the Pork Industry." Peta.org, accessed March 3, 2005, http://www.peta.org.factsheet/files/FactsheetDisplay.asp?ID=119

Pyevich, Caroline. "Sugar and other sweeteners: Do they contain animal products?" *Vegetarian Journal.* Volume XVI, no. 2, March/April 1997; accessed Feb. 25, 2005, http://www.stanford.edu/group/vegan/sweeteners.htm

Robbins, John. *Diet For A New America.* Walpole: Stillpoint, 1987.

Roberts, H.J., M.D. "The Bressler Report." *Sun Sentinel Press;* accessed Feb. 22, 2005, http://www.presidiotex.com/bressler/

"Salts That Heal and Salts That Kill." Curezone.com, accessed March 14, 2005, http://www.curezone.com/foods/saltcure.asp

Savona, Natalie. *The Kitchen Shrink: Foods and Recipes for a Healthy Mind.* London: Duncan Baird, 2003.

Schlosser, Eric. "The Cow Jumped Over the U.S.D.A." *New York Times,* Jan. 2, 2004; accessed March 1, 2005, http://www.commondreams.org/views04/0102-06.htm

Schlosser, Eric. *Fast Food Nation: The Dark Side of the All-American*

Meal. New York: Perennial, 2002.

Severson, Kim. "Sugar coated: We're drowning in high fructose corn syrup. Do the risks go beyond our waistline?" *San Francisco Chronicle* on the Web, Feb. 18, 2004; accessed Feb. 10, 2005, http://www.sfgate.com/cgi-bin/article.cgi?f=/chronicle/ archive/2004/02/18/FDGS24VKMH1.DTL

Simon, Michele. "Dairy Industry Propaganda: Tale of Two Mega-Campaigns." Originally published at Vegan.com, April 1999; accessed Feb. 7, 2005, http://www.informedeating.org/ docs/dairy_industry_propaganda.html

Simon, Michele. "Misery on the Menu: The National School Lunch Program." Originally published in *The Animal's Agenda,* September/October 1998; accessed Feb. 7, 2005, http://www.informedeating.org/docs/misery_on_the_menu.html

Simon, Michele, JD, MPH. "The Politics of Meat and Dairy." Earthsave.org, accessed Jan. 26, 2005, http://wwwearthsave.org/news/polsmd.htm

"Soft Drinks, High-Fructose Corn Syrup Promote Diabetes, Says Study." March 10, 2005; accessed March 15, 2005, http://www.newstarget.com/002584

Squires, Sally. "Sweet but Not So Innocent?" *The Washington Post* on the Web, March 11, 2003; accessed 18 Feb 2005, http://www.washingtonpost.com/ac2/wp-dyn/A8003-2003Mar10?language=printer

Steinman, David. *Diet for a Poisoned Planet: How to Choose Safe Foods for You and Your Family.* New York: Harmony, 1990.

"Sugar Blues." Natural Nutrition, accessed Feb. 2, 2005, http://livrite.com/sugar1.htm

"Surgeon General Asks: Got Bones?" Gotmilk.com, Oct. 26, 2004; accessed March 21, 2005, http://www.gotmilk.com/news/news_035.html

"10 Reasons to Avoid Acidosis." Poly MVA Survivors.com, accessed March 28, 2005, http://polymvasurvivors.com/4corners_coral.html

"Two New Studies Sour Milk's Image." Pcrm.org, Dec. 3, 2004; accessed March 20, 2005, http://www.pcrm.org/news/release041202.html

"Unhealthy link between caffeine and diabetes." CBC Health & Science News, Jan. 9, 2002; accessed Feb. 20, 2005, http://www.cbc.ca/story/science/ national/2002/01/09/caffeine_diabetes020109.html

"The U.S. Food and Drug Administration (FDA) and the glutamate industry." July 12, 2004; accessed Feb. 4, 2005, http://www.truthinlabeling.org/legislators2.html

"USDA Cover-Up of Mad Cow Cases." organicconsumers.org, May 10, 2005; accessed June 1, 2005, http://www.organicconsumers.org/bytes/051005.cfm

"USDA won't stop use of illegal hormones in the veal industry:

cancer rates skyrocket in humans." Jan. 26, 2005; accessed Jan. 27, 2005, http://www.newstarget.com/z0001067.html

U.S. Department Of Agriculture. APIS Veterinary Services. January 2005. "National Animal Identification System: Goal and Visions," accessed March 12, 2005, http://animalid.usda.gov/ nais/about/nais_overview_fact-sheet.shtml

U.S. Department Of Agriculture. "About USDA"; accessed March 12, 2005, http://www.usda.gov/wps/portal/!ut/p/_s.7_0_A/7 _0_1OB?navtype=MA&navid=ABOUT_USDA

U.S. Department of Health and Human Services. "Symptoms Attributed to Aspartame in Complaints Submitted to the FDA." April 20, 1995; accessed Feb. 22, 2005, http://www.presidiotex.com/ aspartame/Facts/92_Symptoms/92_symptoms.html

Van Straten, Michael. *Super Detox.* London: Quadrille, 2003.

"Vegan FAQs." Vegan Action, accessed Jan. 20, 2005, "http://www.vegan.org/FAQs/

"Vegetarian and Vegan Famous Athletes." Veggie.org, accessed March 21, 2005, http://veggie.org/veggie/famous.veg.ath-letes.shtml

Waehner, Paige. "Exercise Bulimia, the New Eating Disorder," accessed March 5, 2005, http://exercise.about.com/cs/exer-cisehealth/ a/exercisebulimia_p.htm

Wangen, Stephen N.D. "Food Allergy Solutions Review." FoodAllergySolutions.com, July 2003; accessed March 28, 2005, http://www.foodallergysolutions.com/food-allergy-news0307.html

Weil, Andrew, M.D. *Natural Health, Natural Medicine.* Boston: Houghton Mifflin, 1998.

Weil, Andrew, M.D. "Does Soy Have a Dark Side?" Dr. Andrew Weil's Self Healing, March 2003; accessed March 15, 2005, http://www.drweilselfhealing.com

Weiss, Suzanne E. *Reader's Digest: Foods that Harm, Foods that Heal: An A-Z Guide to Safe and Healthy Eating.* Pleasantville: The Reader's Digest Association Inc., 1997.

Whitney, Eleanor Noss, and Sharon Rady Rolfes. *Understanding Nutrition,* 8th ed. Belmont: Wadsworth, 1999.

Wijers-Hasegawa, Yumi. "Bayer's GE Crop Herbicide, Glufosinate, Causes Brain Damage." Goldenharvestorganics.com, accessed March 28, 2005, http://www.ghorganics.com/COMMON%20PESTI-CIDE%20CAUSES%20AGGRESSION%20&%20BRAIN%20DAMAGE.htm

Young, Robert O., Ph.D., and Shelley Redford Young. *The pH Miracle: Balance Your Diet, Reclaim Your Health*. New York: Warner, 2002.

Endnotes

1 Steinman, *Diet for a Poisoned Planet,* 166-7.

2 Young, *The pH Miracle: Balance Your Diet,* Reclaim Your Health, 90.

3 Gold, "Formaldehyde Poisoning from Aspartame."

4 Steinman, 190.

5 Ibid., 191.

6 "Caffeine," ecuremelife.com.

7 "Unhealthy link found between caffeine and diabetes," CBC Health & Science News.

8 Young, 51.

9 Ibid., 24-5.

10 Howell, "Why Choose Organic Coffee?"

11 Steinman, 355.

12 Young, 75.

13 Waehner, "Exercise Bulimia, the New Eating Disorder."

14 Pert, *Molecules of Emotion,* 321-22.

15 Whitney and Rolfes, *Understanding Nutrition*, 44

16 Diamond, *Fit for Life*, 65-69.

17 Chandel, "Sweet Poison," The Sunday Tribune Spectrum, tribuneindia.com.

18 "Sugar Blues," Natural Nutrition, livrite.com.

19 Chandel.

20 "Soft Drinks, High-Fructose Corn Syrup Promote Diabetes, Says Study," new-starget.com.

21 Davis, "A Tale of Two Sweeteners: Aspartame & Stevia," suewidemark.net-firms.com.

22 "Natural Sweeteners, Natural Nutrition, livrite.com.

23 Gold, "Common Toxic and Substances to Avoid," holis-ticmed.com.

24 Murray, "How Aspartame Became Legal—The

Timeline," quantumbalancing.com.

[25] Ibid.

[26] Ibid.

[27] "Department of Health and Human Services-Symptoms Attributed to Aspartame in Complaints Submitted to the FDA," U.S. Department of Health and Human Services, presidiotex.com.

[28] Johnson,"Aspartame . . . A Killer!" *The Sunday Express London,* newfrontier.com.

[29] Hasselberger, "Aspartame: RICO Complaint filed Against Nutra-Sweet, ADA, Monsanto," newmediaexplorer.org.

[30] Young, 89.

[31] Gold, "The Bitter Truth about Artificial Sweeteners," truthcampaign.ukf.net.

[32] *Webster's New World Dictionary* (1982), s.v. "saccharin."

[33] Mercola, "The Potential Dangers of Sucralose, vitaminlady.com

[34] Mercola, "Splenda—Here We Go Again," mercola.com.

[35] Mercola, "The Potential Dangers of Sucralose."

[36] Burros, "Splenda's 'Sugar' Claim Unites Odd Couple of Nutrition Wars," *New York Times,* skyhen.org.

[37] Young, 50-51.

[38] Ibid., 14-15.

[39] "10 Reasons To Avoid Acidosis."

[40] Young, 51-52.

[41] Weil, *Natural Health, Natural Medicine,* 27.

[42] Fuhrman, *Eat to Live,* 98.

[43] Ibid., 95.

[44] Robbins, *Diet for a New America,* 290.

[45] Grace, *A Way Out,* 8-9.

[46] Ibid., 8-10.

[47] Steinman, 76.

[48] Brownlee, "The Beef about UTIs."

[49] Steinman, 73.

50 Cousens, *Conscious Eating,*
    433.

51 Ibid., 315.

52 Ibid., 322.

53 Ibid., 313.

54 Wijers-Hasegawa, "Bayer's
    GE Crop Herbicide,
    Glufosinate, Causes Brain
    Damage."

55 Cousens, 438.

56 Steinman, 90.

57 Ibid., 80.

58 "Men's Health Warns of Foods
    You Should Never Eat,"
    Peta.org.

59 Baillie-Hamilton, *The Body
    Restoration Plan,* 36.

60 Ibid., 34-5.

61 "FDA Approved Animal Drug
    Products," FDA 'Green
    Book' section.

62 Mason and Singer, *Animal
    Factories,* 75.

63 "The Latest In Cancer: 'White
    Meat' Linked to Colon
    Cancer," pcrm.org; Singh
    PN, Fraser GE. Dietary risk
    factors for colon cancer in a
    low-risk population. Am J
    Epidem 1998; 148:761-74.

64 Ibid.

65 Robbins, 303.

66 Steinman, 73.

67 Ibid., 313-14.

68 "Fish and Shellfish:
    Contamination Problems
    Preclude Inclusion in the
    Dietary Guidelines for
    Americans," pcrm.org,
    Spring 2004.

69 Weiss, *Reader's Digest: Foods
    that Harm, Foods that Heal,*
    345.

70 Weil, *Natural Health, Natural
    Medicine,* 37.

71 Weil, "Does Soy Have a Dark
    Side?" drandrewweil-
    selfhealing.com.

72 Diamond, *Fit For Life II,* 242.

73 Cousens, 479.

74 "10 Reasons To Avoid
    Acidosis,"
    PolyMVASurvivors.com.

75 Diamond, *Fit For Life II,* 243.

[76] "Milk Sucks," milksucks.com.

[77] Ibid.

[78] Ibid.

[79] Cohen, "The Essence of Betrayal," notmilk.com.

[80] Wangen "Food Allergy Solutions Review," FoodAllergySolutions.com.

[81] "Milk Sucks: Find Out more," milksucks.com.

[82] "Two New Studies Sour Milk's Image," pcrm.org.

[83] Robbins, 150.

[84] Steinman, 131-132.

[85] "Milk Sucks," milksucks.com.

[86] Cousens, 478.

[87] Steinman, 122.

[88] Holford, *The Optimum Nutrition Bible*, 42.

[89] Robbins, 164.

[90] Cousens, 316.

[91] Weiss, 87.

[92] Eisnitz, *Slaughterhouse,* 20, 24-25, 31.

[93] Ibid, 66.

[94] Ibid., 69-70.

[95] Ibid., 126-133.

[96] Ibid., 29.

[97] Ibid., 20, 28-29.

[98] Ibid., 71.

[99] Ibid., 166.

[100] Ibid.

[101] Ibid.

[102] Ibid.

[103] Ibid., front jacket.

[104] Ibid., 124.

[105] Ibid., 82.

[106] Ibid., 125.

[107] Ibid., 87.

[108] Ibid., 84.

[109] Ibid., 91.

[110] Ibid., 93.

[111] Ibid., 130.

[112] Ibid., 132.

[113] Ibid., 132-133.

[114] Ibid., 144-145.

[115] Ibid., 145.

[116] Ibid., 93.

[117] Ibid., 133.

[118] Ibid., 140-141.

[119] Ibid., 172.

[120] Ibid.

[121] Ibid., 173.

[122] Ibid., 174.

[123] Ibid., 175.

[124] Leake, "The rich emotional & intellectual lives of cows."

[125] "The Hidden Lives of Chickens," Peta.org.

[126] "Pigs: Smart Animals at the Mercy of the Pork Industry," Peta.org.

[127] "Fish Feel Pain," Fishinghurts.com.

[128] "Free-Range Eggs and Meat: Conning Consumers?" Peta.org.

[129] "Investigation Reveals Slaughter Horrors at Agriprocessors," Peta.org.

[130] Eisnitz, "Ask the Experts," Peta.org.

[131] Eisnitz, *Slaughterhouse*, 125.

[132] Brown, e-mail.

[133] "Animal Friendly Quotes," Peta.org.

[134] "Everything you need to eat right for your health," Peta.org.

[135] "Factory Farming: Environmental Consequences," Animalalliance.ca.

[136] Cook, "Environmental Hogwash," inthesetimes.com.

[137] Cousens, 442.

[138] Young, 82-3.

[139] Howell, *Enzyme Nutrition*, 4.

[140] Ibid., 4-5.

[141] Cousens, 299.

[142] Ibid., 299.

[143] Ibid., 313.

[144] Ibid., 417.

[145] Holford, 29.

[146] Cousens, 312.

[147] Ibid.

[148] Holford, 41.

[149] Cousens, 587.

[150] "Vegetarian and Vegan Famous Athletes," Veggie.org.

[151] Weil, *Natural Health, Natural Medicine,* 30.

[152] Young, 68.

[153] Whitney and Rolfes, *Understanding Nutrition,* 8th ed., 130-31.

[154] Kamen, *New Facts About Fiber,* 43-85.

[155] Ibid., 14.

[156] Ibid., 10.

[157] Holford, 109.

[158] "About USDA," U.S. Department of Agriculture.

[159] Schlosser, "The Cow Jumped Over the U.S.D.A," *New York Times,* commondreams.org.

[160] Simon, "The Politics of Meat and Dairy," earthsave.org.

[161] Langeland, "Tainted Meat, Tainted Money: Consumer groups decry coziness between government, agribusiness," *Colorado Springs Independent online.*

[162] Schlosser, "The Cow Jumped Over the U.S.D.A."

[163] Ibid.

[164] Ibid.

[165] "National Animal Identification System: Goal and Vision," U.S. Department of Agriculture APIS Veterinary Services.

[166] Ibid.

[167] "USDA Cover-Up of Mad Cow Cases," organic-consumers.org

[168] "USDA won't stop use of illegal hormones in the veal industry: cancer rates skyrocket in humans," newstarget.com.

[169] Nestle, *Food Politics: How the Food Industry Influences Nutrition and Health,* 73.

[170] Ibid.

[171] "Common Dairy Digestive Under-Recognized and Under-Diagnosed in Minorities," Johnson & Johnson.

[172] Simon, "Dairy Industry Propaganda: Tale of Two Mega-Campaigns," origi-

nally published on vegan.com.

[173] "Surgeon General Asks: Got Bones?" gotmilk.com.

[174] Simon, "Dairy Industry Propaganda."

[175] "Surgeon General Asks: Got Bones?"

[176] "About USDA."

[177] Simon, "The Politics of Meat and Dairy."

[178] Simon, "Misery on the Menu: The National School Lunch Program," originally published in *The Animal's Agenda,* informedeating.org.

[179] Schlosser, *Fast Food Nation,* 219-20.

[180] Simon, "Misery on the Menu."

[181] "Food and Nutrition Assistance Programs," Economic Research Service, USDA.gov.

[182] Simon, "The Politics of Meat and Dairy."

[183] Ness, "Organic Food: Outcry Over Rule Changes that Allow More Pesticides, Hormones," *The San Francisco Chronicle,* commondreams.org.

[184] "Organic Industry and Consumers Celebrate USDA Reversal on Non-Food National Organic Standards," The Weston A. Price Foundation, weston-aprice.org.

[185] Harris, "Organic Consumers Association (OCA), the Nation's Largest Organic Consumer Group Denounces Degradation of Organic Food Standards by Congress," about.com.

[186] "Organic Industry and Consumers Celebrate USDA Reversal on Non-Food National Organic Standards."

[187] Krebs, "USDA Accused of Allowing 'Sham' Certifiers to Participate in National organic Program," *The Agribusiness Examiner.*

[188] "OCA and Environmental Groups Sue USDA to

Enforce Strict Standards: Environmental Groups Back Harvey Lawsuit," Organic Business News, organicconsumers.org.

[189] "Nation's Largest Organic Dairy Brand, Horizon, Accused of Violating Organic Standards," The Cornucopia Institute.

[190] Simon, "The Politics of Meat and Dairy."

[191] Green, "Not Milk: The USDA, Monsanto, and the U.S. Dairy Industry," *LiP Magazine.*

[192] Ibid.

[193] "The U.S. Food and Drug Administration (FDA) and the glutamate industry," truthinlabeling.org.

[194] "Food Additives," new-fitness.com.

[195] "Banned as Human Food, StarLink Corn Found in Food Aid," *Environmental News Service.*

[196] Greger, "Rocket Fuel in Milk," Dr.Greger.org.

[197] Ibid.

[198] Cook.

[199] Ibid.

[200] Schlosser, *Fast Food Nation,* 210-214.

[201] Cook.

[202] Barnard, *Breaking the Food Seduction,* 17-19.

[203] Ibid., 20-21.

[204] Ibid., 50-51.

[205] Ibid., 52.

[206] Ibid., 53.

[207] Diamond, *Fit For Life II,* 245.

[208] Barnard, 99-102.

[209] Ibid., 111-14.

[210] Cousens, 231-32.

[211] Van Straten, *Super Detox,* 12.

[212] Cousens, 231-34.

[213] Ibid., 232.

[214] Van Staten, 13.

[215] Cousens, 233.

[216] Ibid., 234.

[217] Ibid., 231.

[218] Mindell, *Earl Mindell's New*

Vitamin Bible, 39-127.

[219] Boschen, "Cycles of the Body," thejuiceguy.com.

[220] Farlow, *Food Additives: A Shopper's Guide To What's Safe & What's Not,* 7-75; "Caring Consumer Guide," Peta.org.

[221] Weil, *Natural Health, Natural Medicine,* 17-18.

[222] Holford, 24.

[223] Farlow, 41-2.

[224] "Salts that Heal and Salts that Kill," curezone.com.

[225] "National Cattlemen's Beef Association Pays for Sadistic Anti-Vegan 'Study,'" vegsource.com.

[226] Myss, *Anatomy of the Spirit,* 53-55.

P.S. Wait! We have a confession to make. We really couldn't care less about being skinny. Don't get scared or upset; you will definitely lose weight if you adopt the *Skinny Bitch* lifestyle. However, our real hope is for you to become healthy. We don't want anyone to be obsessed with getting skinny. When you eat right and exercise, you feel strong and healthy and confident. You start loving your body—not because you lose weight—but because you feel great. It's an inside job. You're finally treating your body like the temple it is.

Comparison is the thief of joy. No matter what we do, most of us will never look like supermodels or celebrities. And accepting that will make our lives a whole lot better. So what if there is only one standard of beauty perpetuated by Hollywood that you don't fit into? Don't buy into that bullshit. Take excellent care of the body you were blessed with, and love, love, love it!

—Rory Freedman and Kim Barnouin

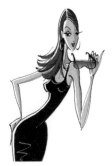